Diverticular Disease of the Colon—
A Deficiency Disease of Western Civilization

Diverticular Disease of the Colon—
A DEFICIENCY DISEASE OF WESTERN CIVILIZATION

by

Neil S. Painter, M.S. (London), F.R.C.S. (England), F.A.C.S.,
D.OBST., R.C.O.G.

Senior Surgeon, The Manor House Hospital, London N.W.11
Hunterian Professor, Royal College of Surgeons of England, 1963
Fellow of the Linnean Society
Fellow of the Harveian Society of London
Honorary Secretary, Section of Surgery,
Royal Society of Medicine, 1975
Fellow of the Zoological Society of London

William Heinemann Medical Books Ltd
London

LSNRNJ

First published 1975

© Neil S. Painter 1975

ISBN 0 433 24660 X

Text set in 11/12 pt Monotype Times New Roman,
printed by letterpress and bound in Great Britain at
The Pitman Press, Bath

To
JOY, RICHARD and MARK

Preface

The purpose of this book is to describe some of the recent advances that have been made in our understanding of colonic physiology and their relation to the causation and to the symptoms of diverticular disease of the colon. In particular, the traditional and current views as to the aetiology and to the pathogenesis of the disease are discussed at length as they form the basis of the modern management of diverticular disease. The conservative treatment of the condition by dietary means is dealt with more fully than are the complications of true inflammatory diverticulitis because the latter have been described many times elsewhere and are dealt with in Bentley Colcock's excellent monograph, 'Diverticular Disease of the Colon'.

Colonoscopy has been mentioned but briefly because, at the present time, it is available only to the few and its advantages and indications have yet to be determined.

The name, 'Diverticular Disease of the Colon' is now used to embrace the time-honoured terms 'diverticulosis' and 'diverticulitis' which date from the days when it was believed that the diverticula were the primary abnormality. It is now known that changes in the behaviour and the structure of the colonic muscle occur before the mucosa herniates and that diverticula are not responsible for symptoms except when they become infected and true inflammatory diverticulitis is present. This modern name for the condition has the advantage of shifting our attention away from the diverticula and directing it towards the changes in the colonic muscle that are so prominent a feature of the disease.

However, I believe that these muscular changes are merely the equivalent of the trabeculation which is seen in the urinary bladder that has had to struggle for years to propel its contents and, consequently, that the thickening and distortion of the muscle is secondary to extra-colonic factors. The historical emergence of this 'new disease' on the clinical scene when taken together with its geographical prevalence leads me to conclude that diverticula are only the outward visible signs of an acquired abnormality caused by our fibre-deficient Western diet.

In the industrialized countries, most foodstuffs have been processed to improve their keeping qualities and to facilitate their transport and many have been refined to make them more palatable so that they can be sold at a greater profit. Consequently, the citizens of these countries eat much more refined sugar and white flour than did their forebears with the result that their intake of plant, and in particular cereal, fibre has diminished dramatically. One object of this book is to show that diverticular disease is a deficiency disease that is due to a diet depleted of fibre. The symptoms of the uncomplicated disease can be relieved or abolished by the addition of cereal fibre in the form of bran to the diet and so there is every hope that it will be possible to prevent the appearance of this disease in succeeding generations by a simple change in our eating habits.

It is hoped that the recognition of diverticulosis coli as a deficiency disease will stimulate research into the causation of the other diseases which also have appeared in the Western world in this century and which I believe are due, at least in part, to the refining of carbohydrates.

February 1975   N.S.P.

Acknowledgements

This book would never have been written had not I benefited from the expert tuition, encouragement and kindness of Dr S. C. Truelove. The pressure studies combined with simultaneous cineradiography which led to the understanding of the pathogenesis of diverticulosis were made in 1961 during the tenure of a research grant which was held while under his supervision at Oxford. This grant was obtained by the efforts of the late Professor P. R. Allison. As a result of this, I received a basic training in clinical research that I would otherwise have missed. The cine-radiographic films were taken by the late Mr Maurice Tuckey, Chief Technician to the Nuffield Institute for Medical Research, Oxford. Dr Kenneth Lumsden, Radiologist to the United Oxford Hospitals, spent many hours assisting me to interpret these films and Professor L. J. Witts gave me facilities in his Nuffield Department of Medicine.

Since then, I have been helped by many people including Dr Basil Morson, Pathologist to St Mark's Hospital and Dr John Madden of St Clare's Hospital, New York, regarding the pathology and the surgical treatment of the disease.

Although the study of the intracolonic pressures had convinced me that the 'low residue diet' is contra-indicated in the treatment of the disease, especially as it is absent in Africans who eat a bulk-forming diet, it was Surgeon Captain T. L. Cleave, R.N., (retired), who convinced me that diverticulosis is only one of many 'modern' diseases that are caused by our over-refined diet. Later, he and Mr Harold Dodd told me of their experiences with millers' bran in the treatment of constipation, with the result that a high-fibre diet has now been used for over seven years at Manor House Hospital where it has been shown that the simple addition of bran will relieve the symptoms of diverticulosis and lessen the need for surgery in the treatment of the disease. Mr Denis Burkitt, Dr Hugh Trowell and Dr Alec

Walker have given their help freely regarding the epidemiology of the disease and its relation to other diseases of civilization. Dr Kenneth Heaton has helped me to design a diet sheet advising patients how to take cereal fibre. Mr Edmund Godding and Mr Harold Godfrey have advised me regarding the properties and dangers of laxatives and bulk-formers.

My thanks are also due to Mr. Norman Tanner for writing the Foreword, Mr Michael Reilly for the chapter on his operation of sigmoid myotomy and Dr Louis Kreel for describing the radiology of the disease. Miss Margaret McLarty and Mr Frank Price drew the diagrams, some of which are published by the kind permission of the editors of the journals in which they first appeared.

Finally, it is a pleasure to thank my colleagues at Manor House Hospital, Mr Anthony Almeida, Dr Kenneth Colebourne, Dr Stewart Reynolds, Dr Florence Telfer, Mr John Barnfather of the Pathological Laboratory and Mrs Sheila Garrod, Superintendent Radiographer, who helped with the transit time studies, together with the pharmacists, the nursing staff and Records Department.

Mrs Joan Rhodes and Mrs Vivienne Dimant assisted my personal secretary, Miss Joan Inglis, who gave invaluable help with the follow-up of patients and typed this manuscript.

I wish to thank Mr Owen R. Evans and Dr Raymond Greene of William Heinemann Medical Books Ltd for their advice and patience in the preparation of this book.

To these and many others, I offer my sincere thanks.

Foreword

NORMAN C. TANNER, M.D., F.R.C.S.,
F.A.C.S.(Hon.), F.R.C.S.I.(Hon.), F.I.C.S.(Hon.)
*Honorary Consultant Surgeon to Charing Cross and
to St James's Hospital, London*

Diverticular disease of the colon remains one of the enigmas of pathology. It is of interest to the physician because of its symptoms, but of paramount concern to the surgeon who has to deal with its complications.

Mr Painter has written perhaps the most outstanding study of colonic diverticulosis and diverticulitis since the classic work of Harold Edwards, and has brought our knowledge of it up to date.

This book will hold the interest of all who read it, family doctors, physicians, surgeons, epidemiologists and even laymen.

In the review of the disease in different countries, emphasis has been rightly placed on diet. This was an emphasis brought very much to the fore in the teaching of the late Professor A. Rendle-Short of Bristol in his studies of the rise of appendicitis and reflected in the writings of Surgeon Captain Cleave (who like myself was one of Rendle-Short's students).

Nevertheless, *every* variation in diet and habit between the diverticulous and nondiverticulous races must be debated. In the Middle East, diverticulosis is almost unknown and yet in some areas a low residue diet is used and constipation is a common complaint. The squatting position is commonly adopted in everyday rest and conversation. Does the squatting position reduce the intra-colonic pressure or even more important increase the ease of gas release through the anus? We look forward to further studies on this subject.

In the meantime, if we wish to study the up-to-date history, the anatomy, the pathology and complications of diverticulosis there can be no better preparation than to read Mr Painter's book, one which has involved years of arduous, honest and unbiased research.

Contents

Contents

Chapter 1

Definitions

A Colonic Diverticulum is, for all practical purposes, a herniation of the colonic mucosa through the muscular wall of the colon and hence diverticular disease is an acquired condition, (Fischer, 1900–1901). True diverticula of the colon containing all coats of the colonic wall have been described, but they may well have been exaggerated haustra (Edel, 1894). Fifield (1927) found no true diverticula in 10,167 consecutive autopsies at the London Hospital (Fig. 1).

The term 'diverticulum' is derived from the Latin 'diverto'

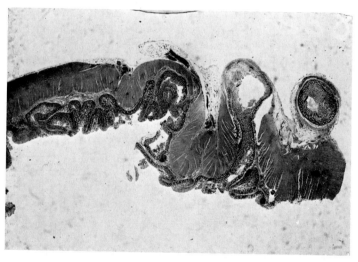

Fig. 1. Longitudinal section of colon bearing diverticula. The colonic wall on the left side of the illustration is apparently normal but it abruptly changed to bowel that is obviously abnormal on the right. The muscle coat on the right is thrown into folds of reduplicated muscle between which the mucosa has herniated to form two diverticula, only one of which has been sectioned so as to show its neck.

The change of structure from the normal to the diseased bowel is sudden and it is not difficult to see why the apparently normal bowel in diverticulosis produces a different pattern of pressures from that part of the bowel that is narrowed and is beset with diverticula (from Painter, 1964).

which means 'I turn aside'. The -*culum* is a diminutive which corresponds to the English—*icle*, as in *follicle* or *cubicle*. So the English equivalent to 'divericulum' is 'divertick' meaning a 'small turning aside' that is a pouch of limited size (Edwards, 1939). The former name is hallowed by official usage although the English 'diverticle' is used colloquially.

Diverticulosis implies that diverticula are present but that they are not inflamed. It was once thought that they did not cause any symptoms unless they were inflamed. This is still probably true but diverticulosis may be *associated* with symptoms as these are caused by some abnormal action of the colonic muscle of which diverticula are only the outward visible sign. Patients with diverticula may complain of symptoms even in the absence of true inflammatory diverticulitis and, furthermore, these symptoms may be cured by changing the diet or by Reilly's operation, and neither of these procedures remove the diverticula. Consequently, it is safer to say that symptoms are associated with diverticulosis as it may well be that they owe their origin to that part of the intestine that is proximal to the colon (Painter 1968 and 1972; Painter, Almeida and Colebourne, 1972).

The term 'diverticulosis' came into being when contrast radiology revealed that diverticula were common and, as the name diverticulitis was already in common use, the word 'diverticulosis' was coined independently by the German-speaking de Quervain, the American J. T. Case and by Sir Ernest Spriggs in England.

Diverticulitis obviously means that diverticula are both present and inflamed. In practice, it usually means that pericolitis is also present as the inflammatory process is not confined to one or more of the mucosal pouches once patients complain of symptoms of sufficient severity to merit this diagnosis. It was once assumed that colonic pain and other abdominal symptoms in patients with diverticulosis were caused by inflammation of the diverticula but it is now realized that excessive segmentation of the colon may cause recurrent pain or colic that is so severe that it may merit sigmoid colectomy. However, when resected sigmoid colons are examined, histological evidence of true inflammatory diverticulitis is often lacking (Morson, 1963). This condition is called *Painful Diverticular Disease*. It causes pain that is usually colicky in character as it is due to intermittent functional obstruction of the colon brought about by excessive segmentation, but it may be so severe that it may be mistaken for left renal colic and morphine or pethidine given for its relief (Painter, 1964 and 1968).

The term *Low Residue Diet* has been used since the nineteen-twenties and, although it may mean different things to those in differing disciplines, to doctors it means that such a diet is, in the main, absorbed by the bowel and consequently it leads to a small quantity of faeces being passed. Most doctors also understand it to mean that pips, seeds, skins and stalks and so-called 'roughage' have been removed from any fruit and vegetables that form part of this diet.

The term *High Residue Diet* implies that the diet contains all those constituents which are not absorbed by the gut so that the stools are large and usually soft, whereas it has a different meaning to some dieticians. In this book, a High Residue Diet is synonymous with a *High Fibre Diet*. This latter term obviously means that the diet contains plenty of fibre. Dietary fibre is difficult to define but it will be seen, when the connection between diet and disease is under consideration, that cereal fibre probably has a special part to play in the physiology of the gastro-intestinal tract.

Chapter 2

The History of Diverticular Disease of the Colon

The diagnosis of diverticulosis depends on the demonstration of diverticula. Until radiological methods of examining the colon became available, the prevalence of diverticula was not realized and only the complications of diverticulitis had attracted attention. The profession became aware of the common occurrence of diverticula only when the radiological demonstration of diverticula had become a routine matter, and only then could the disease be classified and the symptoms and the complications of the condition be differentiated from those caused by other disorders. The changing pattern of the disease and the progress of medicine have divided the story of diverticular disease into six parts.

PART I

COLONIC DIVERTICULA AS A PATHOLOGICAL CURIOSITY

Voigtel (1804) first described these acquired hernia of the large bowel. Fleishman (1815) used the term 'divertikel' to refer to duodenal diverticula found at autopsy and also described single and multiple diverticula of the colon which he found mostly at the mesocolic border. He suggested that they were caused by distension of the gut by food, drink and air. Some have credited Matthew Baillie (1797) with the first description of diverticula but it appears that he described recto-vesical and rectovaginal fistula due to abscesses of the bowel.

Samuel Gross (1845) of Philadelphia described colonic diverticula and illustrated those of the small intestine. 'Sac like tumours . . . are sometimes found in the bowel, caused by protrusion of the mucous and cellular tunics across the muscular fibres, in the same manner as pouches are occasionally formed in the urinary bladder . . . Their number ranges from one to several dozens . . . Professor J. B. S. Jackson of Boston . . . has met with them most frequently in the large bowel, in aged and corpulent persons. Their development seems to depend on some mechanical obstacle to the passage of faecal matter by which the muscular fibres are separated from each other so as to permit the mucous . . . membranes to protrude through the resulting intervals.'

Thus the earliest writers put forward the two theories of the pathogenesis of diverticula. The former believed that passive distension was to blame for their appearance, but the latter was proved right more than a century later when functional obstruction of the colon was shown to cause diverticulosis (Painter, 1962 and 1964).

Rokitansky (1849) described colonic diverticula and their contained faecoliths. Cruveilhier (1849) blamed the hardening of the faeces and straining at stool for their appearance and realized that faecal matter in the mucous pouches might lead to inflammation and to perforation. This complication probably occurred without being recognized at this time as Virchow (1853) described 'chronic adhesive peritonitis' usually with fibrosis that usually affected the sigmoid colon and might be accompanied by abscess formation that was not tubercular in origin.

Bristowe (1854) exhibited a typical case of sigmoid diverticulitis to the Pathological Society of London and described the tendency of the mucosal herniations to enter the appendices epiploica. On microscopic examination, he failed to find muscle fibres covering the pouches and concluded that they were herniations of the mucous membrane. He looked for, but failed to find, any mechanical obstruction of the bowel distal to the diverticula and concluded 'that the cause producing the abnormal condition must have resembled that operating in the case of the sacculated bladder; very likely habitual costiveness may have brought about some of the ill effects which might be expected to follow on actual obstruction'.

Haberschon (1857), physician to Guys' Hospital, described diverticula very accurately in a chapter on constipation contained in what is probably the first textbook of gastro-enterology published in the English language (Lloyd Davies, 1953). However, he did not believe that they produced symptoms or were in any way dangerous. By contrast, Sidney Jones (1859) described vesico-colic fistula due to diverticulitis in a man of sixty-four who noticed faeces in his urine. He complained of abdominal pain and suffered from extravasation of urine to the scrotum, penis and lower abdomen 'from which he rapidly sank'. Autopsy revealed the sigmoid musculature thrown into transverse folds and a diverticulum that had ulcerated into the bladder which contained a calculus. This had caused urinary obstruction and death.

Generalized peritonitis due to diverticulitis was reported by Loomis (1870) according to Dunn and Woolley (1911); he believed that 'infection traversed the wall of the diverticulum without rupture'.

Arbuthnot Lane (1885) found a loop of colon in the sac of a left inguinal hernia at autopsy. This loop had been obstructed by adhesions and Lane noticed that there were no diverticula on the distended part of the gut but that 'the proximal end of the loop was very narrow and presented a double row of sacculi separated by . . . the band of longitudinal muscle fibre'. Dissection of this specimen convinced him that colonic diverticula resembled those seen in the bladder. He noticed that they were to be found only where the muscle wall was thickened and thrown into ridges. He concluded that diverticula were formed by 'vigorous contraction' of the colon on to its contents (Figure 2). He anticipated the views of Morson (1963) and Painter (1962 and 1964) when he realized that diverticulosis was caused by the action of the colonic muscle.

Harrison Cripps (1888) believed that the majority of vesicocolic fistula were more commonly caused by inflammatory mischief than by cancer but, in describing sixty-three cases, he mentioned diverticula only when quoting the example given by Jones (1859).

Thus, diverticula and the complications of diverticulitis were described accurately in the nineteenth century but they remained objects of curiosity. The muscle changes that precede their appearance were recognized and speculation as to the mechanism of their causation was surprisingly prophetic. Nevertheless, it is obvious that diverticulitis, which so commonly causes death, must have been a rare disease at that time or it would have been recognized more frequently at autopsy. The writings of our predecessors have been quoted at length to show that these men, who over a century ago could foretell the findings of modern research, would have recognized the complications of diverticulitis had the disease been common in their day.

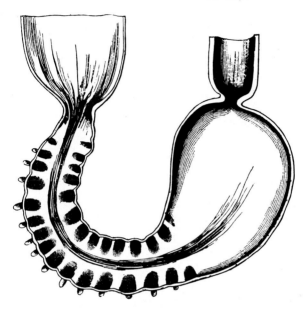

FIG. 2. Arbuthnot Lane's diagram of a sigmoid colon bearing diverticula. He observed that the diverticula were found on the contracted part of the colon and not on the thin distended loops which had resulted from the colon's incarceration in an inguinal hernia. Lane postulated that diverticula were produced by vigorous contraction of the colonic muscle. (Reproduced from Guys' Hospital Reports, by kind permission of the editors.)

PART II

THE RECOGNITION OF DIVERTICULITIS AS A SURGICAL PROBLEM

In 1899, Graser pointed out the potential danger of diverticula in that they became inflamed and gave rise to perisigmoiditis, stenosis and fibrosis of the colon. He warned that peritonitis would follow their perforation. In the next decade, he was proved to be right.

As laparotomy became more commonly practicable, surgeons were surprised by the damage wrought by diverticulitis. In 1903, Bland-Sutton found a piece of straw near to an epiploic appendage which he thought had perforated the colon. He believed that in fat people these appendages caused diverticula by traction and that foreign bodies might penetrate this weak point. He had not been aware of this complication of diverticulitis previously despite being so competent a craftsman that, even in those early days, he could save the life of his patient who had faecal peritonitis. Even Beer (1904) who studied the literature relating to false diverticula, and who collected nineteen reports of complicated diverticulitis, still believed that diverticula seldom caused trouble.

Sir d'Arcy Power (1906) believed in 'pericolic inflammation' which originated in the connective tissue adjoining the sigmoid colon, even though he had the opportunity of seeing four cases of diverticulitis in only a year.

This attitude soon changed. Diverticulitis had entered the clinical arena and was being recognized with increasing certainty. In the same year, Gordinier and Sampson (1906) stated that diverticula caused symptoms more often than had been thought and in the next year Brewer (1907) described abscess formation and peritonitis due to diverticulitis; the latter still thought the condition was rare but caused trouble more often than the literature of the time suggested. Moynihan (1907a and b) described the ability of diverticulitis to cause obstruction and to mimic carcinoma. It is obvious that, at this time, this was still newsworthy as Mayo *et al.* (1907) reported five cases in which diverticulitis with tumour formation had been diagnosed during life; two out of the five patients died of peritonitis following resection, a measure of the hazards attending colonic surgery at that time.

Nevertheless, such diagnoses as 'pericolitis sinistra' and 'torsion of appendices epiploica' lingered on and were still considered respectable. Donaldson (1907) reported abscess formation due to pericolitis in a man of forty-four and believed it was due to some rupture of the mucous membrane due to an unknown cause. Lloyd Roberts (1908) believed that constipation had caused ulceration of the mucosa and abscess formation in the left iliac fossa in one patient, but he did point out that the colon was narrowed and spastic and that diverticula were present. Even as late as 1910, Gordon Taylor and Lakin were at first reluctant to attribute peritonitis to diverticulitis but in retrospect realized that they had dealt with three examples of this problem and suggested that this condition was not so uncommon as was generally thought. In 1908, Dr Maxwell Telling of Leeds described in detail the secondary pathological processes and the symptoms of sigmoid diverticulitis while pointing out that the subject had received 'but scant attention in the literature, especially in England'. It is significant that he said the whole subject was only a few years old and that French, German and American writers also were ascribing increasing importance to the role of diverticula in the causation of disease. There seems no doubt that the condition was a newcomer to the clinical scene and that Telling's paper in the Lancet established diverticulitis as a definite entity in this country.

Patel (1911) collected twenty-eight cases and discredited the 'torsion of appendices epiploica' theory and agreed with Telling that perisigmoiditis was caused by inflamed diverticula. Giffin (1911) reported abscess formation due to a rectal diverticulum and stated that between 1902 and 1910 fifteen operations for diverticulitis had been performed at the Mayo clinic but by 1912 he could review twenty-seven such cases and discuss the differential diagnosis between diverticulitis and carcinoma of the colon.

In 1917, two papers appeared in the British Journal of Surgery which summarized what was known of colonic diverticula and of diverticulitis at that time. Hamilton Drummond described the anatomy of the colon and of the mucosal herniations and their tendency to follow the course of the blood vessels (Fig. 3). Unlike many others, he did not claim that the weakness caused by these vessels was the cause of diverticulosis but concluded that, 'the blood vessels of the normal colon may be said to predispose to sacculi to the same extent as the spermatic cord does to an inguinal hernia'.

In the same year, and in the same journal, Telling and Gruner (1917) published their classic paper on 'Acquired Diverticula, Diverticulitis and Peridiverticulitis of the Large Intestine'. Encouraged by Lord Moynihan, they enlarged on Telling's paper of 1908 and discussed the theories of the causation of the disease as they were surprised to find that only 21% of their patients were constipated. They said that the disease should never be diagnosed under the age of thirty-five. They thought that it was acquired and due to high intra-colonic pressures as did Sir Arthur Keith (1910) who blamed muscle contraction for these postulated pressures and for the hernia. They were

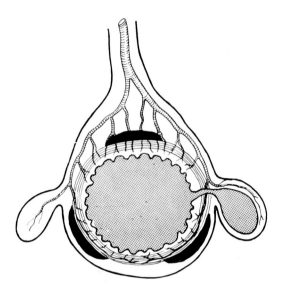

Fɪɢ. 3. Diagram of cross section of human colon in diverticulosis. The colonic lumen is surrounded by a layer of circular muscle that is complete outside which the longitudinal muscle is gathered into three taenia, one of which is at the meso-colic border. The colonic wall is obviously weaker between the taenia. The blood vessels that supply the colon pierce the circular muscle and weaken it further by forming tunnels. It is through these points of least resistance that diverticula in the main emerge. This is the classical diagram of Hamilton Drummond (1917) but Slack (1962 and 1966) has shown that there are two rows of diverticula on each side of the colon.

able to collect no less than 324 examples of diverticulitis from the literature of which 14% had led to stenosis, 28·4% had led to perforation and 19·8% to fistula formation. Not only did they suggest that diet might alter the flora and the speed of the faecal stream but they prophesied that barium x-rays of the sigmoid might well make diagnosis easier. They also advocated resection of the diverticula-bearing gut to avoid future complications.

Their contribution contained all that was known of the disease before radiology became widely used. The disease had changed from a rarity to a common complaint in only twenty years. Dr Maxwell Telling said that he saw his first case in 1899 when he could find nothing about it in the medical writings or anyone who was familiar with it but, by 1908, he could describe the pattern of the disease in detail. Diverticulitis surprised even surgeons of high repute early in the century but by 1920 Sir John Bland-Sutton remarked, 'that in the last ten years acute diverticulitis . . . is recognized with the same certainty as appendicitis. Thus, diverticulitis is a newly-discovered bane of elders.'

PART III

THE DISEASE BECOMES A MEDICAL PROBLEM OF INCREASING MAGNITUDE

Between the two world wars, diverticulosis was found to be a common disorder whose incidence was steadily increasing. The radiological appearances of this new condition were described and its pathological anatomy were investigated in detail. Not surprisingly, there was much speculation as to its aetiology but almost no research was done on this subject. Consequently, the medical management of the disease was founded on theory which was later proved to be incorrect. It was believed at that time that 'roughage' irritated the gut, so a low residue diet became the accepted basis of conservative treatment despite the absence of any evidence that it was of benefit. Similarly, the surgeons of the day were hampered by the technical limitations of colonic surgery. Although they realized that resection afforded the only chance of cure, they were reluctant to operate when anastomosis of the large bowel carried a mortality of up to 25 %, and so surgical intervention was reserved for complications that threatened life.

The changing incidence of diverticulosis is discussed in Chapter 11. By 1923, diverticulitis was sufficiently common to be listed as a cause of death in the Registrar General's reports for England and Wales. This was due in part to the advent of radiology. Haenisch (1912) demonstrated diverticula in the descending colon but it was de Quervain and Spriggs in Europe together with Carman and Case in America who made the barium enema popular. De Quervain (1914) recorded that his assistants diagnosed diverticula first by oral barium and then gave a barium enema to a second patient with acute diverticulitis and this was followed by perforation and peritonitis. Le Wald of New York outlined diverticula by means of a combined opaque meal and enema; his diagnosis was confirmed by subsequent surgery (Abbé, 1914). By 1915, Case had found diverticula thirteen times by x-rays but Carman (1915a and b), who had demonstrated them as early as January 1914, still thought they were uncommon as did Spriggs (1920) who saw diverticula sixteen times in one thousand x-rays.

The term 'diverticulosis', meaning that diverticula were present but were not inflamed or causing symptoms, was proposed by the German-speaking de Quervain (1927) and used independently by Case (1928) and by Sir Ernest Spriggs (Spriggs and Marxer, 1925). By 1924, Judd and Pollock realized that the current statistics were wrong and clinical experience showed that the disease was not rare as one third of positive x-rays at the Mayo Clinic showed diverticula.

In 1925 Sir Ernest Spriggs and his radiographer, Marxer, described the radiological appearances of the disease and discussed its aetiology and treatment. These acute observers recognized that changes occurred in the colon before the actual herniation of the mucosa took place. They called this the 'prediverticular stage' of the disease. It is now thought that this 'stage' represents changes in the colonic musculature which are akin to trabeculation of the urinary bladder (Painter and Burkitt, 1971), but they interpreted it as evidence of 'sigmoiditis' due to the stagnation of faeces in the colon. Consequently, it seemed logical at the time to give liquid paraffin to cleanse the colon and sufficient fruit and vegetables to keep the bowels open easily in the hope of stopping concretions forming in diverticula that might lead to inflammation. They did not advocate a low residue diet any more than did Case (1928) or Mayo (1930) both of whom believed that the colon had to struggle with a low residue diet.

However, by 1930, Slesinger of Guy's Hospital was prohibiting the intake, not only of roughage, pips and seeds, but also of green vegetables. Thus, the low residue diet became the basis of medical treatment (Oschner and Bargen (1935), Willard and Bockus (1936), Brown and Marcley (1937), Edwards (1939)).

Harold Edwards (1934a and b) reported that between 1925 and 1931, 10·8% of barium enemas at Kings College Hospital showed diverticula. He studied the histology of this 'new' disease and demonstrated that before the diverticula appeared the circular muscle was thrown into ridges, when seen on longitudinal section, due to the muscle fibres being gathered into bundles, between which the muscle was extremely thin and the serosa and mucosa came into close relationship. This work was of the greatest importance as it provided a material basis for the changes that had been reported radiologically and, also, for the appearance of diverticula. Edwards suggested that the sigmoid might harbour the highest pressures as it contracted against solid faeces, echoes of Arbuthnot Lane (1888), but as apparatus capable of measuring intra-colonic pressures accurately was not then available, his conclusions were not confirmed until Painter (1962 and 1964) and Arfwiddson (1964) measured these pressures.

Likewise, the surgeons were handicapped by the technology of the time. They knew that successful resection of the colon offered the only hope of cure but colonic anastomosis was still so dangerous that a relieving colostomy was often the only intervention that could be justified (Rankin, 1930; Lockhart-Mummery, 1938). It must be remembered that gastric suction, intravenous therapy and blood transfusion were almost unknown before the last war, and anaesthesia was primitive by modern standards. The contemporary attitude of the profession was summed up by Eggers (1941) who, after describing his experience of eighty-two patients suffering from symptomatic diverticulitis, said that surgery should be reserved for serious complications. Consequently, most patients were given a low residue diet with liquid paraffin in an attempt to prevent the onset of diverticulitis and so the rate of cure for the condition remained extremely low.

PART IV

THE SURGICAL ATTACK ON DIVERTICULITIS

In 1942, Reginald Smithwick published a paper that showed that the dangers attending colonic surgery could be greatly reduced by careful planning. He concluded that defensive surgery achieved little and that a more aggressive attitude would enable the diseased colon to be attacked successfully, and as a result, after the second World War 'pre-emptive' surgery became routine in the treatment of diverticulitis.

He estimated that only between 10 and 20% of patients being treated for the disease ever required some form of surgery and, as the condition was still comparatively rare at that time, no one surgeon's experience would be very great. Therefore, he collected several published series and combined them with the surgical experience of the Massachusetts General Hospital over the previous fifteen years. The following facts emerged from this study.

The complications of acute perforation, abscess and fistula accounted for about 40% of all operations. The mortality from all procedures, including simple colostomy, varied from 9 to 24%, average 17·1%, while no less than one quarter of those treated by primary resection and anastomosis died. Among the fortunate survivors, only 60% were well and about another 10% died of the disease later. Procedures that were lesser than resection were not only ineffective in relieving symptoms but did not even reduce the eventual mortality from diverticulitis. He found, however, that if resection was successful, only 3·7% died later due to further episodes of diverticulitis and over three quarters remained well and symptom free.

He concluded that, 'the outlook of patients with severe forms of diverticulitis is not very bright'. To say the least, this was an understatement.

He argued that, as diverticulitis was localized to only one defined part of the sigmoid colon, resection was feasible.

Attempts to exteriorize the affected bowel, with or without colostomy, gave poor results, and although the Mickulicz type of resection was safe, it was not always technically possible. He noticed that a more extensive resection gave better results than did a more limited excision. Leakage from the anastomosis was a major cause of death and neither an accompanying or a preliminary caecostomy lessened the incidence of this complication. However, if a preliminary colostomy had been performed and the inflammatory process allowed to settle for between three and six months, the subsequent resection and anastomosis were relatively safe.

His plea for planned resection before serious complications occurred is a milestone in the story of the disease. It came at a time when few doctors would subject patients to colonic surgery for a benign disease because of the risks involved. At the same time, many realized that the quality of life of patients with recurrent diverticulitis or with a permanent colostomy was far from satisfactory and so many surgeons were sympathetic to the view that a planned resection of the sigmoid was preferable to lethal complications at some future date—always providing that the operation could be made safe.

Fortunately, Smithwick's advocacy of more aggressive surgery coincided with the advent of the antibiotics, advances in anaesthesia and blood transfusion and in supportive therapy generally. As a result, elective resection became a standard procedure in the next decade. The credit for this is mainly due to American surgeons as most of the reports of this era came from the U.S.A. The author believes that there may have been a good reason for this. Diverticulitis had increased in prevalence in England until 1939 when the death rate from the disease became static. This may well have been due to the less refined wartime diet forced on the British people, which provided them with extra fibre and helped to prevent the disease. No such change occurred in America and there the disease continued to cause an increasing problem which had to be tackled.

There is no doubt that it was tackled. Smithwick's claim that staged resection was the safest procedure was echoed by Morton (1946). By 1947, Pemberton, Black and Maino examined and restated the role of surgery in diverticulitis. They found that at the Mayo Clinic between the years 1908 and 1940 even simple colostomy killed one in twenty patients, but after this date its mortality had dropped to only 1%. The death rate from resection in the corresponding period had fallen from 17% to 5%. They stressed that if a proximal colostomy had been fashioned it should never be closed unless the distal diseased bowel had been resected as in twenty-nine cases where closure preceded resection no less than twenty patients had suffered subsequently from recurrent diverticulitis. Having shown that both colostomy and resection now could be carried out with an acceptable risk, they argued that the indications for resection should be broadened so as to prevent the possibility of lethal complications at some future date. They attributed the improved results of surgery to the sulpha drugs and antibiotics, in the main, while admitting that both surgical technique and after-care had also advanced with the setting up of a special unit for colon surgery.

Boyden (1950) reported that Dr Thomas Joyce of Portland, Oregon, had attacked the disease by resection between 1929 and 1944 in twenty-seven cases and almost always without a preliminary colostomy. This had lowered morbidity and so Boyden favoured early resection if only because of the difficulty in distinguishing between diverticulitis and carcinoma. He believed that a colostomy should always be established in the presence of obstruction and that resection should follow after only two to nine weeks. He also reported nine successful primary resections performed without a colostomy.

It was soon realized that this more radical surgery cured symptoms and lowered morbidity. This led to the adoption of elective resection, preferably as the procedure of choice. By 1950, Mayo and Blunt could report that resection used in the correction of vesico-colic fistula only carried a 6·5% mortality. Lloyd-Davies (1953) favoured early resection especially when obstruction had occurred because in about one half of such cases it was impossible to exclude the presence of cancer.

The good results of staged resection almost inevitably encouraged others to perform a one-stage resection without colostomy. When successful, this lessened the time in hospital and the risks attending more than one operation. Judd and Mears (1953) treated recurrent diverticulitis, fistula, abscess and even obstruction at one operation with only one death due to concurrent disease; while others suited the type of operation to the problem that confronted them using procedures involving one, two or three stages. The changes that occurred in the attitude of surgeons can be gauged by the report of Waugh and Walt (1957), namely that 30% of 320 patients with diverticulitis had been treated by a one-stage resection from 1945 to 1954; primary resection was safe as only one of ninety-three patients had died. McCune and Iovine (1957) favoured one stage resection when the disease was in remission but stressed that they would add a colostomy if the extent of the disease prevented them obtaining normal bowel for anastomosis; this accords with the recommendation of Welch, Allen and Donaldson (1953) that over 20 cm. of bowel should be resected. The virtues of primary resection were also extolled by Strenger (1957) and Waugh and Walt (1959), while in England, Lloyd-Davies (1953) advocated earlier resection and pointed out that even the most complicated cases, that necessitated long and difficult operations, could be cured by more aggressive surgery. Todd (1955) remarked that resection was safe and that surgeons were still too reluctant to advise radical surgery.

Thus the treatment of diverticulitis changed dramatically after the second World War. Previously, surgeons had only operated for complications when life was threatened. Often this meant that they did too little and too late. Once resection was shown to be safe, especially if all the thickened bowel was removed, elective surgery became commoner. At first advanced cases with complications were tackled successfully and then, as confidence increased, recurrent pain in the left iliac fossa became an indication for sigmoid colectomy. This was performed in the belief that the patient had recurrent diverticulitis and as less diseased colons were resected, more and more one-stage operations were performed. This represented a great advance and by 1958 Barborka concluded that elective resection was not only the treatment of choice but should be performed even earlier. One-stage sigmoid colectomy had become so commonplace that he felt it necessary to say that when operating for perforation or obstruction, preliminary colostomy was mandatory.

This sudden swing to primary anastomosis was not without danger. Disruption of a colonic anastomosis is a serious complication that may be fatal. The distal colon is the most treacherous part of the gut to anastomose and most surgeons have experienced or seen the serious complications that may follow leakage from an anastomosis in the pelvic colon. Such disasters are seldom published and it is certain that a number of patients have died due to disruption of an anastomosis, following one-stage resection, which had been performed because the operation had become fashionable in the surgical literature. These patients would have survived for many years if a simple colostomy had been fashioned, whether or not a curative operation had been performed later. While colonic surgeons can keep the mortality of sigmoid resection low, this is not the case with those who are less experienced or less interested in this branch of surgery. Consequently, Colcock (1951 and 1971) has warned quite rightly against being over-confident when dealing with a disease which so often calls for the greatest skill and judgement. There is no disgrace in performing a colostomy or in staging procedures, to suit the patient or the extent of the disease process. Discretion is the better part of valour when the patient's life is at stake. There is no doubt that the surgery of diverticulitis is theoretically simple but often technically difficult (Thompson, 1959).

By 1960, elective resection, with or without colostomy, had

become the procedure of choice in diverticulitis. The methods employed are still a matter for discussion. In the preceding twenty years the disease had become one of the major problems of surgery, but the majority of patients were still looked after by their physicians who gave them laxatives and a low residue diet. The fourth phase of the story of the disease ended when the physiology of the colon became understood better and the pathology of the disease was examined by Morson (1963). This led to further improvements in the medical and surgical management of what was soon to be called 'diverticular disease of the colon'.

PART V

THE RECOGNITION OF THE ROLE OF THE COLONIC MUSCLE IN THE PATHOGENESIS OF DIVERTICULA

The abnormality of the muscle coat that had been blamed for the disease as long ago as 1845 by Gross and later by Harold Edwards was shown to be responsible for the herniation of the mucosa by Painter (1962 and 1964) in England and by Arfwidsson (1964) in Sweden. This led to the recognition of the part played by segmentation in colonic physiology in the production of the localized pressures that cause diverticulosis. These advances ushered in the fifth phase of our understanding of the disease process.

At the same time Morson (1963) studied the pathological changes in 155 specimens resected at St Mark's Hospital with a pre-operative diagnosis of 'diverticulitis'. He found that only in one third of them was there histological evidence of sufficient inflammation to justify this diagnosis or to account for the severe pain that had led to major surgery. He showed that the thickening of the colonic muscle was a constant feature in his specimens and he also reported that he could not demonstrate the presence of diverticula in some specimens even though the sigmoid colon had been resected for 'diverticulitis'. Likewise Arfwidsson studied the typical changes in the muscle and confirmed that in the 'pre-diverticular state' the thickening of the circular and longitudinal muscle occurred before the diverticula appeared and that these changes were accompanied by the ability of the altered colon to produce higher pressures than the normal colon. He came to the same conclusion as Morson, namely that the muscle changes preceded the actual herniation of the mucosa while Painter and his colleagues (1965) recorded abnormally high pressures in the immediate vicinity of a single diverticulum in the sigmoid, thus showing that the abnormal pressure response was present in a very early stage of the disease.

The muscle thickening, and its radiological appearances, were described by Williams (1963) who showed that the classical radiological signs of 'diverticulitis' cannot be explained on the basis of inflammation but only by a primary fault in the action of the colonic muscle which could be present in the absence of diverticula.

Painter (1964) suggested that the pain of so-called 'acute diverticulitis' was often the colic of intermittent functional obstruction brought about by excessive segmentation of the colon and was not due to the inflammation of diverticula. He pointed out that the urinary bladder produces severe pain, even in the absence of infection, when its outflow is obstructed, and that a similar state of affairs might apply to the segments of the colon whose outflow is occluded on each side by excessive segmentation. The term 'Painful Diverticular Disease' was used by Painter (1968) to describe this colic which waxes and wanes with a rapidity that is inconsistent with the onset and resolution of an inflammatory process.

These observations led to a reappraisal of the term 'diverticulitis'; the term means that an inflammatory process is present and should no longer be used to describe pain of colonic origin.

Thus the attention of the profession shifted from the actual diverticula towards the colonic muscle. The present author believes that the changes seen in the muscle of the colon in diverticulosis represent 'trabeculation' of the colon and that this corresponds to that seen in the urinary bladder whose outflow has been partially obstructed for many years.

The thickening of the sigmoid muscle is often very localized and Reilly (1964, 1966) realized that this pathological change was often the only abnormality present and so he questioned whether it was necessary to resect an otherwise normal sigmoid colon just because its lumen was narrowed. He devised the operation of sigmoid myotomy in which the muscle is divided longitudinally down to the sub-mucosa as an alternative to resection. The operation is similar to a Ramstedt's or Heller's procedure and in selected cases is as effective as resection but entails less risk. The division of the circular muscle fibres restores the lumen of the bowel, and reduces the intracolonic pressures. The fact that Reilly's operation relieves symptoms shows that they are due to muscular activity and not to the diverticula which remain *in situ* at the end of the operation.

Thus in the last few years modern technology has made it possible to show that abnormal activity of the colonic muscle is responsible, not only for the production of diverticula, but also for the symptoms that had been attributed previously to 'diverticulitis'. This knowledge was applied by Reilly who devised his 'physiological' operation of sigmoid myotomy. The term 'diverticular disease of the colon' came into use once it was realized that the diverticula were secondary to some disorder of colonic motility. The pathogenesis of the condition was now understood but the aetiology of diverticulosis still remained a mystery.

PART VI

DIVERTICULOSIS AS A DEFICIENCY DISEASE

The appearance of the disease and its emergence as a major medical problem, which have been described, leave little doubt that it is a 'new' disease. Evidence is accumulating that it is the result of the changes which occurred in our diet towards the end of the last century and which altered the environment of the colon. The geographical distribution of the disease reveals that it is rare or unknown to this very day in the rural African and Asian and in all countries where traditional eating habits have not changed. The disease is unknown where the diet contains plenty of cereal fibre but it has become the commonest disorder of the colon in those countries whose food is processed and refined (Cleave, Campbell and Painter, 1969; Painter, 1970; Painter and Burkitt, 1971).

The connection between dietary fibre and bowel behaviour has been demonstrated and discussed by Burkitt, Walker and Painter (1972) and by others. Where the diet is fibre deficient the intestinal transit time is prolonged and the daily weight of stool passed is low. Conversely, the inclusion of plenty of cereal fibre in food produces large soft stools that traverse the bowel rapidly. The replacement of the bran fibre which is missing from our modern diet has been shown to relieve 85% of the symptoms of uncomplicated diverticular disease (Painter, Almeida and Colebourne, 1972).

At the present time, it appears that the aetiology of diverticular disease is linked to fibre-deficiency. Consequently, like scurvy, the disease should be preventible. One purpose of the book is to draw attention to the fact that if the citizens of this country would return to a less refined diet containing the natural amount of fibre, there is every reason to believe that our children might not suffer from the disease or from its companions, appendicitis and cancer of the colon.

Chapter 3

Pathological Anatomy

(1) INTRODUCTION

A colonic diverticulum is, for practical purposes, a herniation of the mucosa through the muscular wall of the colon.

The colonic wall consists of a mucous membrane of which the muscularis mucosa is a part, separated from the deep muscle layers by loose elastic connective tissue. The inner of the two muscle layers consists of fasciculi of circular fibres which form a continuous tube around the bowel. Outside this is the longitudinal muscle coat, which also forms a continuous sheath around the bowel, but is very much thinner than the circular muscle (Lineback, 1925; Hamilton, 1946). It is mainly concentrated into three bands of taenia coli. In the sigmoid region one of these lies at the mesocolic border of the colon and the other two are anti-mesocolic; all three are relatively broader in this region and so the interval between them is narrow. The three taenia fuse into one coat at the recto-sigmoid junction which is usually about six inches above the peritoneal reflection.

The taenia coli are about one sixth shorter than the rest of the intestine to which they belong and, consequently, are credited with causing the shortening of the colon that bunches it into sacculations or haustra. The taenia and the circular muscle are joined by bundles of muscle fibres passing between them. Hence the ability of each layer to act independently is limited. The circular muscle is anchored to the taenia and it would appear that this gives it a fixed base upon which it can contract and demarcate the colon into clefts or haustra.

Between the taenia, the colonic wall is obviously weaker as it consists mainly of circular muscle and this muscle is further weakened by the segmental blood vessels which pierce it at regular intervals. These vessels are derived from the marginal artery (Griffiths, 1961) and they pass outside the mesocolic taenia and give off two large branches on each side of the colon. These branches pass through the muscle coat in the interval between the meso-colic taenia and the anti-mesocolic taenia. They then tunnel through the circular muscle to supply the colonic wall at its anti-mesocolic border (Fig. 3). Diverticula commonly emerge along the track charted by these lateral vessels so that they are found in two rows on each side of the affected colon; the close relationship of diverticula to these vessels has been demonstrated by Noer (1955) and Slack (1962), both of whom injected the colonic arteries with radio-opaque material and used x-rays to show their intra-mural anatomy (Fig. 4). Slack must be credited for drawing the profession's

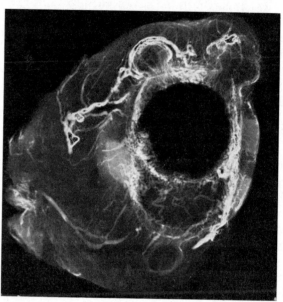

FIG. 4. The relationship of diverticula to the colonic blood vessels. This shows a transverse section of a colon whose arteries had been injected with barium. Two diverticula are clearly shown on the left. Their close relationship with the blood vessels is obvious. The author is indebted to Mr W. W. Slack for this photograph.

attention to the existence of two rows of diverticula on each side of the colon. Prior to his work, the classical diagram of Hamilton Drummond (1917) had been accepted as accurate and this showed only one diverticulum on the side of each segment.

The tunnel formed by the blood vessels is a point of potential weakness and this anatomical arrangement has been blamed for diverticulosis. However, it is obvious that the structure of the colon is common both to those with the disease and to those who do not develop diverticula and to the very young. These vessels only determine the commonest site of diverticula, but they are not responsible for their appearance. The blood vessels bear to diverticula the same relationship as does the spermatic cord to an inguinal hernia (Drummond, 1917). Furthermore, diverticula do occur on other parts of the colon's circumference where they are only related to minute intramural blood vessels (David, 1933; Watts and Marcus, 1964; Fleischner *et al.*, 1964).

The intimate relationship of diverticula to the segmental blood vessels is less apparent in the advanced stages of the disease as diverticula may burrow between the muscle of the colon or coalesce with each other so that the architecture of the colon is distorted (Cohen, Cunningham and Snierson, 1957).

Early in their development diverticula, like other hernia, are reducible and consequently they may not be found in post-mortem specimens without the greatest difficulty. At first, their covering may contain a few muscle fibres but these soon atrophy and diverticula then consist of sacs of mucous membrane covered only by connective tissue and the serosa. They then have not the power to expel faeces and often their necks are narrowed by the circular muscle, so that their contained faeces become inspissated. In this way faecoliths form which may cause inflammation, presumably by irritating the mucous membrane. As a result, diverticula may become fixed by fibrous scar tissue so that they are no longer reducible.

The structure of the muscular components of the healthy colon and of the colon that is beset with diverticula has been studied very thoroughly by many workers, but no congenital abnormality that would account for the appearance of diverticula has ever been demonstrated convincingly (Edwards, 1954). However, the normal colonic muscle is not of uniform thickness. Poirier and Charpey (1914) described the folds between the colonic haustra and stated that the circular muscle in these folds is reinforced and is augmented in its amount. They suggested that these full thickness folds could act as baffles and slow the passage of faecal material. David (1937) agreed with their findings after examining the sigmoid colons of old people and he described areas where the muscle coat was thinner and also diverticula that were not related to blood vessels. Torsoli, Crucioli and Young (1969) measured the thickness of the muscle in the colonic folds and found that it was significantly greater than that in the muscle coat between the folds; they also showed that the colonic musculature is thickest in the sigmoid region. These authors appear to have described structural features that might account for the segmentation which occurs in the living colon (Painter, 1962; 1964; Painter *et al.*, 1965), but Pace and Williams (1969) failed to demonstrate any anatomical basis for the intersegmental contraction rings which are so clearly seen radiologically when the normal or the diseased colon is segmenting. The role of the circular muscle and of the taenia is not yet fully understood and this makes the interpretation of the pathological anatomy of the diseased colon difficult.

(2) THE PATHOLOGICAL ANATOMY OF ESTABLISHED DIVERTICULOSIS

The most striking feature of established diverticular disease is seen in the sigmoid colon. The muscle coat is greatly thickened and palpation reveals that often this thickening begins abruptly at the recto-sigmoid junction and above this point the bowel has been converted into a rigid tube with a narrowed lumen (Figs. 1 and 5). Often this thickening is limited to a few inches of the sigmoid but its upper limit may not be so well defined and the upper sigmoid may gradually diminish in thickness so that it blends with the proximal colon. The taenia coli are thick and sometimes so hard that they have an almost cartilaginous consistency. The circular muscle is thick and has a corrugated appearance which Sir Arthur Keith (1910) likened to the bellows of a concertina. He deduced, albeit from a fixed specimen, that this appearance was due to a sustained contraction of the taenia which had caused the circular muscle to bunch into folds which narrowed the colonic lumen.

In between these corrugations of reduplicated circular muscle, the mouths of diverticula may be found as they penetrate the bowel wall between the haustra often to be covered by the pericolic fat (Fig. 6). Sometimes no diverticula but only a tendency to sacculation is found between these folds which are covered by mucous membrane. These circular muscle folds and their mucosal covering are not continuous around the whole circumference of the bowel wall but are often semi-circular ridges of muscle confined to the area between the mesocolic and

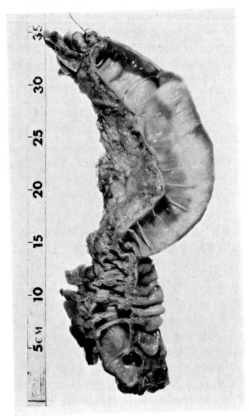

Fig. 5. The macroscopic appearances of diverticular disease of the colon. The specimen is 45 cm. long and consists of the descending and sigmoid colon. There is extensive diverticulosis with thickening and corrugation of the bowel wall in the sigmoid region but no active inflammation. Some of the diverticula contain faecoliths. The change between the apparently normal colon and the diseased segments of the bowel is abrupt.

(Photographs and report by courtesy of Dr Basil Morson.)

antimesocolic taenia. In between them, the colonic mucosa may appear to be trabeculated in a manner similar to that seen in the urinary bladder that has had to struggle for many years against a partially obstructed outlet (Morson, 1963). These semi-circular folds may interdigitate (Fig. 7) and each consists of two layers of circular muscle so closely in contact that they appear to be fused together.

The degree of muscular thickening in diverticular disease is variable but it is always greatest in the sigmoid and is never seen

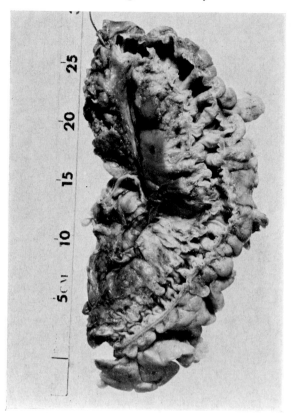

FIG. 6. Diverticular disease of the colon; macroscopic appearances. The specimen shows a colon resected for diverticular disease. Fig. 6a shows the narrowed sigmoid with mucosal and muscular folds. The muscle is thickened but no evidence of inflammation was found on histological examination.

to the same degree in other parts of the colon although slight degrees of thickening, which accentuate the haustra may be found in the ascending and in the transverse colon.

The disease is also distinguished by the apparently redundant mucosa which is often gathered into folds which further contribute to the stenosis of the colonic lumen which has been brought about by the infolding of the circular muscle which has been described. Morson (1963) found it difficult to pass a fine probe through the lumen of a resected sigmoid afflicted by the condition and believes that this redundancy of the colonic mucosa must be a reflection of the extreme shortening of the

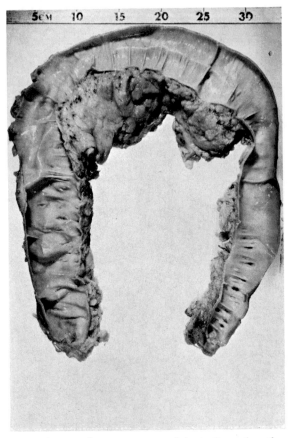

Fɪɢ. 6b shows the ascending, transverse and descending colon; the mouths of diverticula can be clearly seen but the proximal colon does not show the muscle thickening that is so typical of diverticular disease affecting the sigmoid region.

However, sections taken from the proximal colon showed muscular gaps with hyperplastic changes in the overlying mucosa which are typical of the initial changes of the disease process.

(Photographs and report by courtesy of Dr Basil Morson.)

bowel that has resulted from some abnormal and sustained contraction of its muscle.

Often the sigmoid colon is laden with fat to a much greater extent than is the rest of the colon. This was once thought to be the result of recurrent 'diverticulitis', or due to the tendency of corpulent subjects to get diverticulosis. This is not the case as obesity has been discarded as a causative factor in the disease and two thirds of such sigmoids resected for 'diverticulitis' show

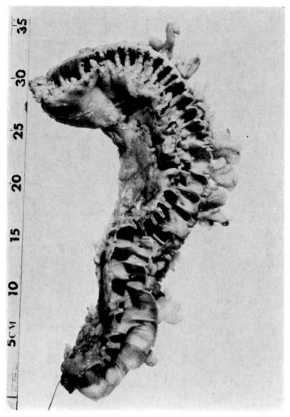

FIG. 7. A sigmoid colon resected for 'diverticulitis'. The specimen is 35 cm. long and shows a sigmoid colon whose wall was greatly thickened. Its muscular folds narrowed the lumen and interdigitated. Histological examination revealed no evidence of inflammation and so the episodes of severe colic which had led to operation were probably caused by intermittent functional obstruction due to contractions of the abnormal colonic muscle.

(Photograph and report by courtesy of Dr Basil Morson.)

no significant evidence of any past inflammation. This apparent excess of pericolic and mesocolic fat is probably due to shortening of the sigmoid which brings the appendices epiploica nearer together (Morson, 1963).

Histologically, it is impossible to say with any degree of certainty that the muscle thickening is due to hypertrophy or to hyperplasia. The nerves and ganglia of Auerbach's and Meisner's plexuses appear to be seen somewhat more frequently in the sigmoid but, again, this could be due to contraction although

Painter (1967) has suggested that the sigmoid has a special nerve supply because it has a special function. Arfwidsson (1964) believes that this thickening of the muscle is the result of hypertrophy similar to that seen in the urinary bladder, a view shared by Lane (1888). Arfwidsson counted the nuclei of the muscle cells and measured their size, and found that the density of nuclei in the thickened sigmoid was less than in the normal sigmoid and this strongly supports the view that the muscle changes found in diverticular disease represent hypertrophy as a similar state of affairs is seen in the hypertrophied left ventricle that accompanies aortic stenosis. On the other hand, Slack (1962; 1969) attempted to determine the number of cells in normal muscle and in the thickened muscle by measuring the DNA content and concluded that the increased muscle thickness was due not to hypertrophy but to either hyperplasia of the muscle cells or to longitudinal contraction of the bowel wall. He argued, like Arfwidsson and Morson, that this thickening is not the result of inflammation, but is the result of some disorder of function.

There is no doubt that, as regards most of the colon, Slack is right in saying that diverticula may be present without any muscle thickening (Fig 6a and b), but in the sigmoid region, which causes most clinical problems, most authorities agree that the muscle thickens and becomes thrown into ridges before diverticula appear. Hughes (1969) considers that the sigmoid is abnormal if its circular muscle is 1·8 mm. or more in thickness and he found colons with thickened muscle and stout muscle bands extending two thirds of the way round the colon in specimens which bore no diverticula. Like Morson (1963) and Arfwidsson (1964) he reported that the muscle abnormality that is so typical of the disease can be present even in the absence of diverticula while Williams (1967) used the term, 'Diverticular Disease of the Colon without Diverticula'. These findings suggest that the structure of the sigmoid alters before diverticula appear much in the same way as the urinary bladder becomes trabeculated long before vesical diverticula develop.

Hughes (1970) investigated the shape of the lumen of the distal colon by giving polysiloxane enemas to patients while in the erect position. These set to a soft consistency within about four minutes and are then evacuated by the patient. This method yields beautiful casts of the rectum, colon and diverticula.

Hughes described three types of abnormality. Type 1 casts showed deep indentations caused by muscular bands with diverticula between the bands. These changes were localized, beginning on average 33 cm. (range 28·5–48 cm.) from the anal margin and continuing upward for a distance of about 12 cm. (average 6–20 cm.). The site of these changes correspond to the localized thickening of the sigmoid that is palpated at operation which Painter (1967) has suggested may result from some special function of the sigmoid colon. Hughes' Type II abnormality consists of four or five curves in the lower sigmoid which can occur separately or just below a Type I deformity and, finally, he described a third type of abnormality in which deep impressions were present on the cast only on one side of the bowel and usually in the concavity of the recto-sigmoid curve. The significance of these three patterns is not yet known nor is it certain whether they represent different forms of the disease. It is possible that they are manifestations of differing stages of the disease process, but only further work will elucidate this point.

THE 'PREDIVERTICULAR STATE' AND THE HISTOLOGICAL CHANGES IN THE COLON THAT PRECEDE THE APPEARANCE OF DIVERTICULA

Spriggs and Marxer (1925, 1927) coined the term 'Prediverticular State' to denote the radiological changes which they observed in colons and in which 'the normal segmentation of the bowel is absent, being replaced by a ragged outline of little convex irregularities'. These appearances have also been called, 'saw toothed', 'serrated edge', 'pallisade' or 'ripple border' by subsequent writers to describe the sigmoid which appears to have contracted in length so that it resembles a concertina. These changes precede the actual appearance of diverticula as Spriggs and Marxer rightly concluded although they believed that they were caused by infection due to the stagnation of faeces in the sigmoid, a theory that has since been discounted.

Edwards (1939) believed that 'each tooth of the saw edge is a diverticulum'. Painter (1962) using cineradiography demonstrated that often it is almost impossible to distinguish radiologically between the apex of a narrow segment and a diverticulum although they may be differentiated on occasion by the administration of certain drugs. The term 'prediverticular state', strictly speaking, describes a colon, or part of a colon, whose haustra are very close together and which has all the attributes of the colon in diverticulosis except that no diverticula have been demonstrated with certainty at the time of examination.

The histological basis for these x-ray appearances has intrigued many investigators but I believe that they were explained by the work of Harold Edwards (1934a and b; 1939). Edwards endeavoured to elucidate the cause of diverticulosis by studying sections of the colon in various stages in the development of the disease process. He showed quite clearly that long before the herniation of the mucosa took place, the circular muscle was of uneven thickness being gathered into 'hillocks' (that is, bundles or circular muscle seen in cross section, Fig. 8). Between these strong strands of circular muscle were gaps where the muscular component of the colonic wall was absent with the result that the mucosa and serosa were in close approximation and there was no solid barrier of tissue to prevent any raised intracolonic pressure driving the mucosa through the circular muscle. He believed that 'irregular spasm' of the circular muscle caused the muscle fibres of the circular muscle to become alternately hypertrophic and atrophic. Edwards proposed that sustained spasm of the muscularis propria acting on its contents generated the pressure which forced the mucosa between the gaps that separated the bundles of circular muscle, and he blamed constipation and the use of purgatives for this irregular muscle spasm.

The present author believes that his work is of supreme importance as it provides histological proof of the differing thickness, and consequently the strength, of the circular muscle that heralds the advent of diverticulosis. Even before diverticula appear, the circular muscle is no longer a sheet of evenly distributed fibres of equal strength because its fibres have gathered together into thick bands which, while they can contract vigorously, cannot concurrently surround the bowel continuously. Consequently, gaps appear between the circular strands and here the muscle coat is weakened sometimes to such an extent that it is absent so that it cannot withstand the intraluminal pressures produced by neighbouring bands of hypertrophied muscle. His work has since been confirmed by others including Conway and Hitzrot (1931), Morson (1963), Fleischner, Ming and Henken (1964); Williams (1967) and Hughes (1964) and also by Arfwidsson (1964) who studied the sigmoid both

Fig. 8a

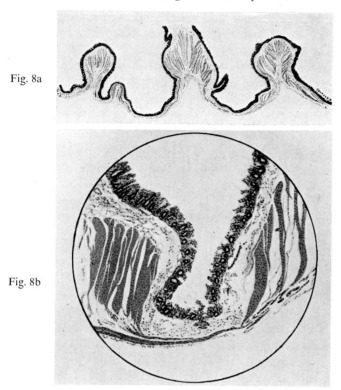

Fig. 8b

FIGS. 8a and 8b. The muscle abnormality in the 'pre-diverticular state'. Fig. 8a is a drawing showing how the circular muscle, when viewed in cross section, is thrown into ridges between which it is thinner. Fig. 8b shows a higher magnification of the same portion of the bowel wall. It will be seen that the mucosa and serosa are in close approximation and there is little to stop the mucosa from herniating between the muscle fibre.

(From Edwards 1939, reproduced by kind permission of the author and the publishers, John Wright and Son, Bristol.)

radiologically and histologically and, at the same time, measured the intra-sigmoid pressures in the 'prediverticular state' and showed that hypertrophy of the sigmoid muscle and pressure changes occur before the mucosa herniates.

Once Harold Edwards had shown that the circular muscle varied in thickness before diverticula appeared, it became easy to understand how the colonic muscle can produce intraluminal pressures which it cannot withstand. The physical basis for the understanding of this apparent paradox is crucial to the pathogenesis of colonic diverticula. This process may be illustrated quite simply by squeezing mud in the hand. As a fist is made the mud, which is almost incompressible, escapes between the fingers. The fingers represent the thickened bands of circular muscle which, in attempting to compress the contents of the colon, force the mucosa through the gaps in the circular muscle.

THE DISTRIBUTION OF DIVERTICULA

Colonic diverticula are not found equally in all parts of the large intestine. Edwards (1939) studied 179 barium enemas all of which showed diverticula and recorded that the disease process affected the sigmoid in 91% of them. He reported that the sigmoid alone was affected in 94 patients, the sigmoid and descending colon in 38 patients, the sigmoid, descending and transverse colon in 18 patients and in 13 patients the whole colon was beset with diverticula. His experience is similar to that of most investigators in the Western countries. Since the time of Sir Ernest Spriggs, the sigmoid has been known to be the site of election of diverticulosis. Recently, in Australia, Hughes (1969) found that the sigmoid bore diverticula in 99% of 90 diseased colons while in a contemporary British series the sigmoid was affected in 443 out of 461 cases, 96% (Parks, 1969). In Hawaiian Japanese, the right side of the colon is the common site of diverticulitis; the reason for this is unknown (Stemmerman, 1970).

It has been said that the sigmoid colon is most affected by the disease because it is the narrowest part of the colon and because it harbours the firmest faeces with the result that it has to generate higher pressures than the rest of the colon. Among others, Connell (1961), Reilly (1966) and Painter (1967) have suggested that the sigmoid has a special function in that it is involved in faecal continence and that this may have some bearing on the fact that it is the commonest site of colonic diverticula.

THE STRENGTH OF THE COLONIC WALL IN DIVERTICULAR DISEASE

No evidence has ever been produced to show that diverticulosis is due to any congenital weakness of the colon, but it seems that the muscle of the colon is normal at birth and changes later.

The historical emergence of the disease in the economically developed countries and its appearance in differing ethnic groups who adopt their way of life indirectly confirms this statement and supports the view that the colon is damaged by some adverse factor in its environment.

The changes in the muscle that are typical of the prediverticular state are probably due to hypertrophy (Arfwidsson, 1964) and this may well be caused by the colon having to overwork over many years as it copes with the residue of our modern abnormal diet (Painter and Burkitt, 1971). At first sight, the thickened diseased colon appears to be stronger than the normal colon but obviously it is not as it cannot prevent the herniation of the mucosa. Edwards' demonstration of the varying thickness of the colonic wall provides anatomical evidence which suggests that diverticular disease weakens the colon, but proof of this in the living colon was lacking until quite recently.

Parks and Connell (1969a and b) measured the ability of the normal sigmoid to withstand a distending force. They placed a balloon in the sigmoid colon of normal subjects and of those affected by the disease and then distended the balloon step by step with 20 ml. increments of water at body temperature. As the balloon increased in volume up to 120 ml., the tension in the balloon and hence in the normal bowel wall steadily rose up to a pressure of about 43 cm. of water. However, when diseased sigmoids were studied this was not the case; the tension rose until the balloon contained about 40 ml. of water but further distension of the balloon even up to 120 ml. did not result in the tension rising above about 25 cm. of water. They concluded that the sigmoid which was beset with diverticula is less able to withstand a stretching force than is the normal bowel. Their experiments on living human subjects showed that in diverticulosis the colonic muscle has been weakened, a fact that had previously been deduced only from the study of dead tissues.

Later Parks (1970a and b) investigated the prediverticular state. He took advantage of the fact that when the sigmoid has been resected for diverticulitis, the descending colon is anastomosed to the rectum. This enables this part of the bowel to be reached by the sigmoidoscope so that its ability to withstand distension can be studied by the means already described. He found that the behaviour of this part of the bowel, which was free of diverticula, did not differ significantly from normal as judged by motility studies but that its reaction to stretch resembled that of the diverticula-bearing sigmoid. The tension in the balloon and the bowel rose to 32 cm. of water as the balloon was inflated with 80 ml. of water but further filling of the balloon up to 120 ml. did not elicit any corresponding increase in the tension of the bowel wall. Parks considered that this demonstrated that, even in segments which did not bear diverticula, some muscle abnormality preceded the appearance of diverticula.

CONCLUSION

The most constant feature of diverticular disease is the thickening of the colonic muscle. This not only accompanies the presence of diverticula but precedes their appearance. This is especially true of the sigmoid region which is the commonest site of the disease in the Western world.

At first sight, the thickened colon would appear to be stronger but this is not the case. Closer inspection reveals that its muscle coat is uneven in thickness and that it consists of bundles of muscle fibres bunched together between which there are gaps where the muscle may be absent and through which the mucosa herniates.

It must, however, be remembered that diverticula can be present in the proximal colon where the muscle remains thin (Fig. 6a and b). This suggests that the aetiology of diverticula of the sigmoid may be different from that of diverticula in the rest of the colon.

The appearances resemble the changes that are typical of the urinary bladder in chronic prostatic obstruction. When it is remembered that the colon functions as a series of 'little bladders' whose outflow becomes partially obstructed during segmentation (Chapter 10), it seems probable that the thickening of the colon which is seen in diverticular disease represents 'trabeculation' of the colonic muscle resulting from excessive segmentation.

Chapter 4

The Radiology of Diverticular Disease
Louis Kreel, MD FRCP FFR

The emergence of diverticular disease as a common condition in the middle aged and elderly in affluent societies has resulted not only in its more frequent recognition, but also in a re-defining of basic terms.

In early years clinicians and radiologists were confident in their ability to distinguish diverticulosis and diverticulitis. This is no longer so. The spiky, narrowed and concertina'd sigmoid colon is now not considered to be a manifestation of inflammatory disease but of over-action of circular muscle. Inflammatory disease of the colon associated with diverticular formation is thought of in terms of pericolic abscess (Fig. 9) and sinus

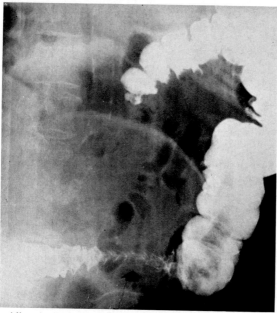

FIG. 9. True 'diverticulitis', which is in fact a pericolic abscess causing a narrowed segment. The mucosal pattern is still visible within it and the ends are funnelled. Note partially filled diverticula in transverse colon.

tracks (Fig. 10). The true 'diverticulitis' or inflammation of a solitary diverticulum only occasionally produces specific radiological features enabling such a specific diagnosis to be made. Hence the insistence on the non-specific term of diverticular disease.

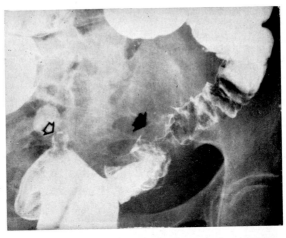

Fig. 10. Diverticular disease with a pericolic abscess and a parallel track (black arrow).

The radiological aspects can be divided into different parts, firstly there is the recognition of diverticula as such and the appearance of circular muscle contraction in the sigmoid region, which is a simple matter (Fig. 11). Secondly, there are the signs which result from the complications associated with this condition. Then there are those signs which depend upon the trapping of opaque substances within diverticula, whether contrast agents or ingested foreign bodies. The most recent radiological contribution is the demonstration of bleeding from a diverticulum by mesenteric angiography and in the context of gastro-intestinal haemorrhage, the relationship between bleeding and the barium enema will also be mentioned, as well as the role of colonoscopy in its diagnosis.

THE CHEST RADIOGRAPH

Only rarely will the chest film show signs resulting from diverticular disease, but because of its age distribution and

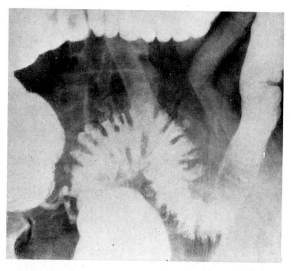

FIG. 11. The appearance previously designated as diverticulitis with marked interdigitating muscle contraction and diverticula protruding from the pockets between. Neither the clinical picture nor these radiological appearances can be correlated with inflammation on histological examination. Hence the modern designation of 'diverticular disease'.

because of the possibility of surgery, it is recommended as a routine in all such patients. Cardiac enlargement must be noted, and as there is the ever-present possibility of colonic carcinoma, metastases must be excluded. In this respect, a raised right hemi-diaphragm is important as a manifestation of an enlarged liver due to tumour infiltration. A pneumoperitoneum resulting from a perforated diverticulum is best seen on an erect chest film.

THE PLAIN FILM OF THE ABDOMEN

Because colonic gas does not accumulate in diverticula, this condition cannot be shown on the plain abdominal film without the use of contrast agents. There is, however, one variety of diverticulum which can be seen by virtue of gas accumulation within it. This is the congenital giant diverticulum of the sigmoid colon which on the plain film appears as a large rounded collection of gas rising out of the pelvis in the region of the left iliac fossa. This entity can also be shown on a barium enema, but the radiological features on the plain film are virtually patho-gnomonic.

It is well recognized that small metallic foreign bodies may become trapped in colonic diverticula, thus indicating their presence. This is particularly so with lead shot used for wild game. The demonstration of these small round opacities on the radiograph indicates not only the anatomical diagnosis but also the social class of the patient.

Similarly, diverticula are shown following a barium meal examination (Fig. 12). The barium becomes trapped in the

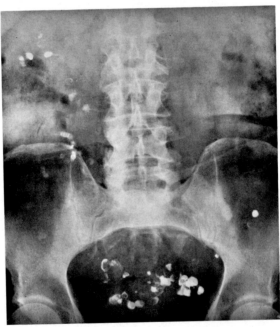

FIG. 12. Barium trapped in diverticula shown on a plain film taken two weeks after a barium meal. Barium can also be seen in the appendix.

diverticula and may remain there for months. Small, rounded dense opacities, especially in the sigmoid region, are thus commonly seen in radiological practice in this country where a film is taken between one week and two months after a barium examination. Even the contrast medium after an oral chole-cystogram will occasionally show up diverticula in this way. Uncommonly, a faecolith in a diverticulum is demonstrated on a plain film due to its calcium content. This occurs particularly on the right side with diverticula of the ascending colon.

The plain film features of obstruction and perforation can be caused by diverticular disease. It is important to remember that, when such radiological signs are seen in the elderly, they are commonly due to this disease and not necessarily a manifestation of malignancy.

Chronic colonic obstruction due to diverticular disease almost invariably occurs in the sigmoid region. This is usually associate with an 'incompetent' ileo-colic sphincter, so that there is distension and fluid levels in both colon and small bowel. The gas patterns indicating whether it is small or large bowel are best seen on the supine film (Fig. 13), whereas the fluid levels are visualized on the erect film. Perforation from diverticular disease may occur either intra-peritoneally or retro-peritoneally, producing markedly differing clinical and radiological manifestations.

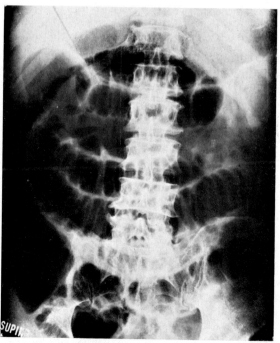

FIG. 13a. A supine film showing distended small bowel in the centre of the abdomen and colon at the periphery, indicating a large bowel obstruction.

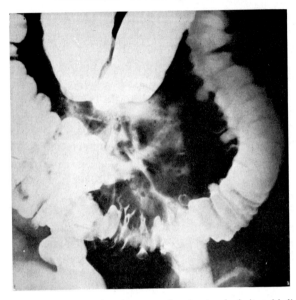

FIG. 13b. Barium enema in the same case showing marked sigmoid diverticular disease.

Free peritoneal perforation usually occurs from a diverticulum of the ascending colon and is seen as gas under the diaphragm in the erect film. If there is sufficient gas, it can also be recognized on the supine film. The actual wall of small bowel or transverse colon will be seen by virtue of gas, both within its lumen and in the peritoneal cavity.

Retroperitoneal perforation is far more serious and far more difficult to recognize. It most frequently occurs from a diverticulum of the sigmoid colon. The clinical manifestations of pain and stiffness around the left hip joint has its radiological counterpart in the presence of multiple small rounded gas shadows in the soft tissues around the left hip. In fact, the most common non-surgical or non-traumatic cause of soft tissue gas in this region is due to a perforated sigmoid diverticulum, and of course signifies impending gas gangrene unless promptly recognized and treated.

Retroperitoneal gas may not only pass downwards towards the left hip following perforation, but also often passes upwards. The soft tissue planes are delineated by gas bubbles which show up the psoas shadows, the peri-renal spaces, and may outline the supra-renals and accumulates below the diaphragm. This produces a characteristic appearance but may, unfortunately, be overlooked because of the overlying small bowel and colon.

Pneumaturia is a well recognized complication of sigmoid diverticular disease. This can be recognized on the plain film as gas in the bladder outlining it on the supine film, or producing a fluid level on the erect view. This gas not infrequently passes up the ureters to the pelvis and calyces, which are outlined as contrast negative shadows. Although this appearance is patho-gnomonic, it can largely be hidden by bowel shadows and then requires a high index of suspicion for its detection.

THE BARIUM EXAMINATION

The technique of the barium enema has altered radically in the last decade. The double contrast method is now practised in most large centres. This, however, has not changed the patterns of recognition of diverticular disease which still depends upon two basic signs. The first is the demonstration of the parallel linear impressions of the contracted circular muscle and the other is the demonstration of the diverticula (Fig. 14). The radiologist is concerned not only with these aspects, but also

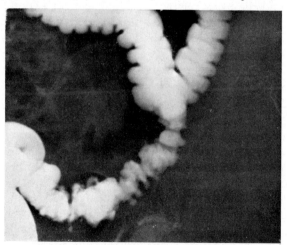

FIG. 14. Typical barium filled sigmoid colon with a moderate degree of diverticular disease. The parallel linear impression of the circular muscle are seen as filling defects between the diverticular-containing pouches of colon.

with the demonstration of any of the complications and the exclusion of associated or incidental diseases, especially carcinoma (Fig. 15).

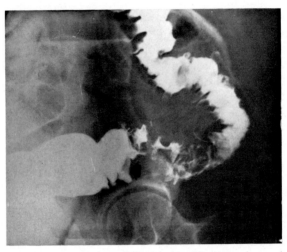

FIG. 15. Carcinoma in a region of diverticular disease causing a shouldering effect and loss of the mucosal pattern in the narrowed segment.

No special preparation is used for cases with diverticular disease and the usual regime of a fluid diet for two days prior to the morning of the examination is recommended, together with the usual laxative. Should contractions of the circular muscle of the sigmoid region greatly impede the flow of barium or raise difficulties in interpretation, intravenous Buscopan can be given during the course of the procedure. Particular attention must be paid to excluding the presence of carcinoma and not being content with ascribing the symptoms to the easily demonstrable diverticula present.

In the sigmoid region, the narrowing due to contraction of the interdigitating circular muscle varies from slight to marked. In the early stages it appears as thick, transverse, parallel half shadowing, the margin of the colon being spiky. This appearance has been called the pre-diverticular stage, and even though no diverticula are visible, it is now recognized that this represents the earliest phase of the disease (Fig. 16). It is, however, of considerable theoretical interest that this appearance occurs only in the sigmoid region, whereas diverticula are found in all

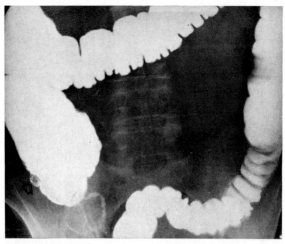

FIG. 16a. Early phase of diverticular disease in the sigmoid colon with marked parallel linear indentations due to the interdigitating thickened bands of circular muscle. There is also a solitary diverticulum at the caecum and a carcinomatous polyp in the descending colon.

parts of the colon and even occasionally in the terminal ileum. Why this muscle contraction should precede diverticula in the sigmoid region and not be demonstrable in the other parts of the colon or in the terminal ileum (Fig. 17) has, as yet, not been explained.

Alternating and interdigitating semicircular bands of smooth muscle produce marked indentations of the barium column. This ultimately produces not just a saw-tooth appearance but more of a zig-zag or see-saw effect, and diverticula formation is usually obvious and gross (Fig. 18). Even at this stage the colonic lumen can be widened by anti-spasmodics such as intravenous Buscopan and by the air insufflation of a double contrast enema.

It was this late appearance which was previously designated as diverticulitis and has now been shown to be independent of any inflammation but due to muscle contraction and hypertrophy. Occasionally, marked intermittent contractions occur in the descending colon, but these are more like peristaltic or stripping waves causing a narrowed segment with a clearly definable mucosal pattern from the margins of which diverticula can be seen protruding.

The herniations of mucosa and submucosa between the muscle layers producing the diverticula are most clearly demonstrated

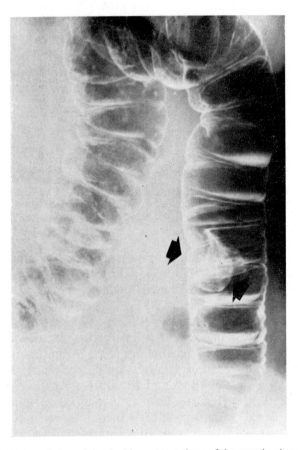

FIG. 16b. Enlarged view of the double contrast phase of the examination showing the carcinomatous polyp.

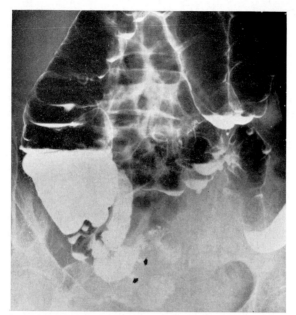

FIG. 17a. Scattered diverticula of the colon, and there are also diverticula on the terminal ileum.

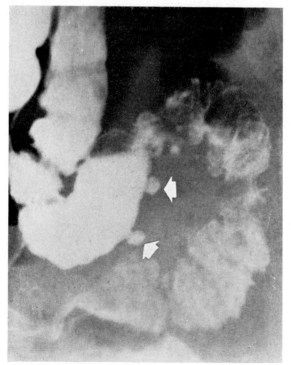

FIG. 17b. Enlarged view of the terminal ileum showing the diverticula. Note that in the terminal ileum and ascending colon the diverticula are *not* associated with muscle contraction.

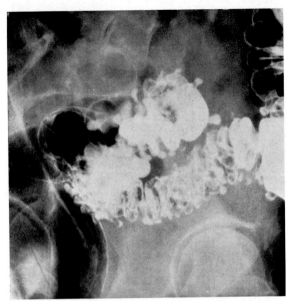

Fig. 18a. Gross diverticular disease of the colon.

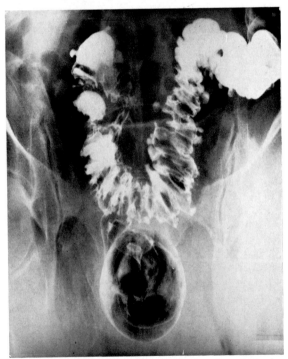

Fig. 18b. The Hampton or modified Chasser–Lapine view which gives a clearer picture of the sigmoid region, showing the zig-zag pattern of gross diverticular disease.

when seen on the edge of the colon. They vary in size from 3 mm. to 3 cm. (Fig. 19) and are mostly well rounded. When completely filled with barium they have a uniform density, but the barium may only outline the periphery of the diverticulum which contains impacted faeces. If the barium partially fills the neck and base of such a faeces-filled diverticulum it produces a 'wine glass' appearance and if only the stem fills it will look like a spike or thorn. Frequently, however, diverticula are superimposed on the colon shadow. They may be mistaken for polyps

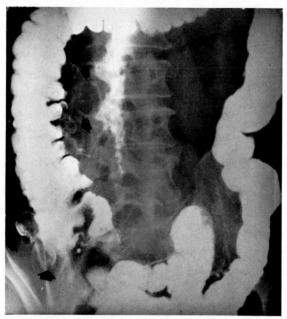

Fig. 19. Large diverticula on the ascending colon with relative sparing of the sigmoid and descending colon.

and the most accurate way to distinguish the two conditions is by obtaining a view at right angles. Diverticula of course protrude from the margin, whereas polyps will always be seen within the margin. Should it not be possible to obtain a view at right angles, the final diagnosis will probably come from sigmoidoscopy or colonoscopy, but the detailed analysis of the appearance of the circular contrast shadow may also be helpful. With a diverticulum, the outer margin of the circular shadow is sharp and the barium shadow is blurred inwards, whereas with

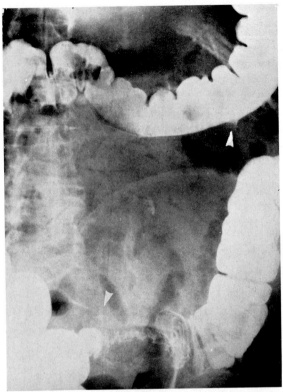

FIG. 20a. Pericolic abscess due to diverticular disease.

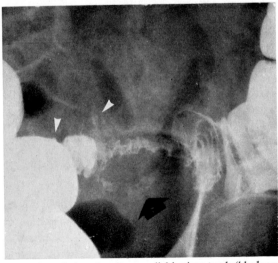

FIG. 20b. Enlarged view showing parallel barium track (black arrow).

a polyp the inner margin of the circular shadow is sharp and the barium shadow fades away outwards.

Whilst diverticular disease is easily recognized on a barium enema, the exact diagnosis of a narrowed segment is more demanding. It may be said that this is in any case academic as an organically narrowed segment will require surgery and the diagnosis will then be established at subsequent histology. Usually, however, surgeons request such information prior to operation and, not uncommonly, even the patient wishes to be informed. Wherever possible, therefore, the distinction between a benign stricture and a malignant one must be attempted on the barium examination. Furthermore, the possibility of a carcinoma being present within an area of diverticular disease must always be borne in mind. The benign stricture of diverticular disease is almost invariably due to a peridiverticular abscess. The mucosal pattern within the narrowed segment remains visible, its ends taper and not infrequently there is also a parallel track of barium at the site of the perforation (Fig. 20). A somewhat similar appearance can occur in Crohn's disease; however in this condition the stricture is usually longer, rose thorn ulcers are present and further lesions may be present elsewhere in the colon or in the small bowel, particularly at the terminal ileum.

Carcinoma in an area of diverticular disease may also produce an extra-luminal track, but the mucosal pattern is lost at the narrowed segment and shouldering becomes visible (Fig. 21). If any doubt exists endoscopy or surgery will, of course, be undertaken. Carcinoma must also be excluded in the rest of the colon. Whereas the double contrast examination makes little difference to its accuracy in the diagnosis of diverticular disease as such, it does however aid considerably in excluding early carcinoma in the rest of the colon, or in confirming a suspected lesion seen on the barium-filled colon.

The suspicious gross changes caused by diverticular disease and its complications are common and easily recognized. However, local perforations or peri-diverticulitis can produce signs on the barium enema which can be extremely difficult to visualize. The small irregular fleck or streak lying adjacent to the colonic margin represents minimal extravasation from a diverticulum. Such a localized perforation may also lead to a bilobed indentation of the margin of the colon with the amputated neck of the diverticulum forming a dimple in its centre. A

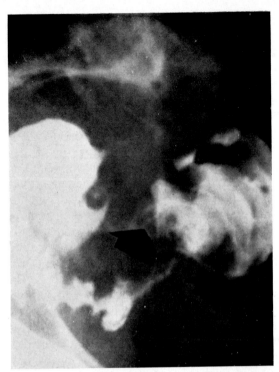

FIG. 21. Shouldering effect of a carcinoma within an area of diverticular disease

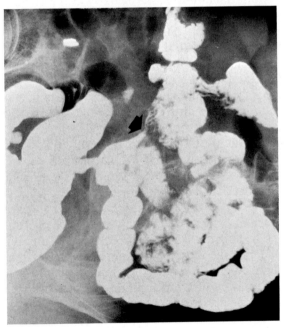

FIG. 22a. Fistula into small bowel seen on a barium enema.

localized extrinsic defect shown best on the distended colon and particularly with the double contrast technique can easily be overlooked. True focal diverticulitis may lead to pointing and distortion of a diverticulum which is best shown by comparison with a previous examination.

Attention is drawn to these minimal radiological signs as they may help to explain episodes of acute pain and tenderness, transient fever and leucocytosis which otherwise will go undiagnosed.

The fistulous complications of diverticular disease are often recognizable on the plain film, as has been mentioned previously. However, these are best shown by barium enema examination and can be recognized by the flow of the barium into small bowel (Fig. 22), bladder, uterus or vagina. The exact delineation

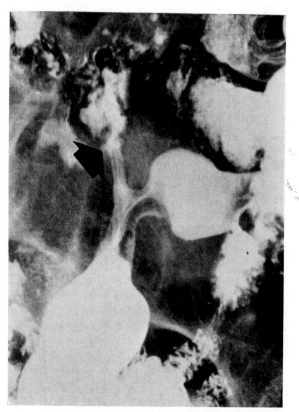

FIG. 22b. Enlarged view showing elongated diverticulum at the site of the fistula formation between sigmoid colon and jejunum.

of the connection is important as it aids surgical localization greatly, and also helps to define the underlying pathology. The stretched neck of the diverticulum may be recognized as well as the mucosal pattern within it, thus distinguishing it from a carcinomatous fistula or Crohn's disease. The adjacent bowel is also often quite normal in appearance in diverticular disease.

Diverticular disease, being a common entity, will not infrequently be found in association with other diseases, particularly in the elderly. This is particularly true of carcinoma, whether occurring with the early pre-diverticular type (Fig. 23) or the late phase. Ischaemic colitis can completely transform the appearance of diverticular disease, so that the colon appears as a narrow, rigid tube with an occasional diverticulum still visible (Fig. 24).

MESENTERIC ANGIOGRAPHY

Gastro-intestinal haemorrhage from colonic diverticula can present a challenging diagnostic and therapeutic problem. The site of this bleeding cannot usually be determined from a barium enema or at laparotomy. It has now been demonstrated that, be selective arteriography this can be done, provided bleeding is occurring at a rate of more than 0·5 ml. per minute, and this appears to be a valuable additional diagnostic method.

With the aid of pre-shaped opaque catheters, image intensification and television monitoring, it has become a relatively simple matter to carry out this procedure. The newer non-toxic arteriographic contrast agents have now made this entirely safe.

Most bleeding diverticula of the colon are in the ascending part, and therefore selective catheterization of the superior mesenteric artery is undertaken for its demonstration. On angiography the site of bleeding is shown by the extravascular accumulation of contrast medium in a confined space. This is demonstrated in the venous or late phase of the examination. Particular stress must be placed on two points; firstly, prior barium examinations will preclude angiography because of the obscuring contrast medium, and secondly, angiography will only produce a positive result in the active phase of bleeding.

It has also been demonstrated that gastro-intestinal haemorrhage can be controlled by intermittent local intra-arterial infusion of pitressin or the injection of blood clot. It thus

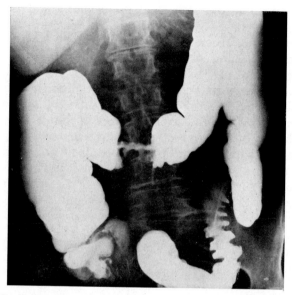

FIG. 23. Early diverticular disease (pre-diverticular stage) in the sigmoid with a carcinoma of the transverse colon.

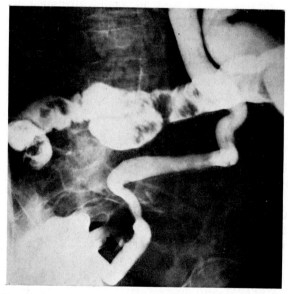

FIG. 24. Diverticulum of the sigmoid colon in a case with ischaemic colitis of the descending and sigmoid regions.

becomes possible to combine both the diagnostic and therapeutic benefits of angiography by using it in this way.

The bleeding from a colonic diverticulum has also been stopped by a barium enema. There is, however, no way of telling which particular diverticulum is the source of the haemorrhage, or indeed if the haemorrhage is coming from a diverticulum, by this examination. Nor can one assume that the source of the haemorrhage is from a diverticulum, even though these have been shown. In the event of continuing haemorrhage, residual barium would obscure the field for subsequent arteriography.

It is therefore recommended that, in the assessment of active colonic haemorrhage angiography must take precedence and performed as an emergency. A barium enema can then be done at a later stage if necessary. There is now in addition, the possibility of the use of colonoscopy to localize the source of such haemorrhage. While this is not available at the moment in all centres, it probably will be in the near future.

Other Investigations.

Bladder and vaginal fistulae and sinuses may require further definition either because these have been shown on an enema examination or have not been adequately demonstrated. These sinus tracks or fistulae can often be more clearly shown by micturating cystourethography, balloon vaginography or sinography.

SUMMARY AND CONCLUSIONS

The newer concepts associated with diverticular disease are now widely accepted. Radiologists should be particularly conversant with these as the diagnosis is primarily radiological.

While the narrowing due to muscle contraction and the diverticula are easily recognized, the complications may require more meticulous attention. This applies particularly to the minimal signs of local perforation. Associated carcinoma is common and must not be overlooked, especially when present within an area narrowed by diverticular disease.

The recent advances in angiography can also be applied to diverticular disease, as can colonoscopy. This adds a further dimension to the management of this disease and will, it is hoped, be available to many more centres in the near future.

REFERENCES

BERANBAUM, S. L., ZAUSNER, J. and LANE, B. (1972). 'Diverticular Disease of the Right Colon'. *Am. J. Roent.* **115**, 334–348.

FLEISCHNER, F. G. and MING, S.-C. (1965). 'Revised Concepts on Diverticular Disease of the Colon—Part II'. *Radiology* **84**, 559–608.

FLEISCHNER, F. G. (1967). *Diverticular Disease and the Irritable Colon Syndrome Alimentary Tract Roentgenology*, Vol. II: 784–810 C. V. Mosby Company, Saint Louis.

GUISTRA, P. E., ROOT, J. A. and KILLORAN, P. J. (1972). 'Rectal Diverticulitis with Perforation'. *Radiology* **105**, 23–4.

LEWIS, E. E. and SCHNUG, G. E. (1972). 'Importance of Angiography in the Management of Massive Haemorrhage from Colonic Diverticula'. *Am. J. Surg.* **124**, 573–580.

MORSON, B. C. (1963). 'The Muscle Abnormality in Diverticular Disease of the Sigmoid Colon'. *Brit. J. Rad.* **36**, 385–392.

WILLIAMS, I. (1963). 'Changing Emphasis in Diverticular Disease of the Colon'. *Brit. J. Rad.* **36**, 393–406.

Chapter 5

The Incidence of Diverticular Disease in the Sexes and in the Young

(1) INTRODUCTION

Diverticulosis is a 'new' disease that has only been recognized in the Western nations in the last seventy years. Consequently, most of the statements made in this chapter refer to the populations of these countries. This is because the disease is still rare in the developing nations of Africa and Asia and has only recently appeared in Japan. It is obvious that as the prevalence of the disease is changing, any statistics concerning the incidence of the disease refer only to the particular population that has been studied and to that population only at the date of investigation. The various methods of determining the prevalence of diverticulosis are discussed in Chapter 11, together with what is known of the incidence of the disease throughout the world at the present time. The influence of sex on this incidence and the rarity of the disease in children and young people are the subjects of this chapter.

(2) THE SEX INCIDENCE OF DIVERTICULAR DISEASE

This appears to be changing as men were once thought to be twice as prone to the disease as were women (Telling and Gruner, 1917; Mayo, 1930; Oschner and Bargen, 1955; Brown and Marcley, 1937); but Morton (1946), Smith (1951), Fagin (1955), Horner (1958) and Kohler (1963) noticed no difference in the sex incidence of the disease. Kocour (1937) in America, found that females, whether white or coloured, were the more prone to the disease. Grout (1949) found that in England nine women were affected for every seven men. Both Patterson (1951) and Greene (1957) in America reported that 60% of diverticulitis was seen in women. The crude death rate per million in England and Wales shows that nowadays more women die from diverticulitis than do men (Fig. 58). This change in the sex incidence is too big to be accounted for by the greater number of women now living in the older age groups, and some unrecognized factor appears to be at work. It is possible that this change is due to the fact that, in the Western world, more women are constipated than men (Avery Jones and Godding, 1971). The desire to stay slim may have discouraged women from eating bread, and hence cereal fibre, which they believe is fattening. However, it must be remembered that these remarks apply to Europe and North America for in Japan, where the disease has appeared in recent years, diverticulosis still seems to be commoner in men and tends to affect the right side of the colon (Stemmerman and Yatani, 1973).

(3) COLONIC DIVERTICULA IN CHILDREN AND YOUNG PEOPLE

Diverticulosis is an acquired disease of the second half of life, being usually seen after the age of forty. This is what would be expected if it is caused by our modern diet and, as food becomes more refined, it is not surprising that in recent years diverticula have been found with increasing frequency in patients under this age and even in young people in their twenties. However, ever since the disease first attracted attention, there have been reports of diverticula appearing very early in life. If these reports are correct, such diverticula can hardly be attributed to the prolonged effect of our abnormal diet on a congenitally normal colon, but whether these cases would stand up to critical investigation by present standards is questionable.

Hartwell and Cecil (1910) thought that congenital and acquired diverticula were indistinguishable and propounded the view that diverticula were congenital and only lost their muscle coat later. From the study of five infants' colons fixed in formalin they claimed that they had found evidence of a congenital weakness in the colon's musculature. They believed that they had demonstrated two diverticula in a six-year-old boy who died of an infectious disease and one in a girl of ten who succumbed to meningitis. Like Turner (1920) and Buie (1939) they believed that a congenital factor was responsible for diverticula that appeared in the young. Bearse (1939 and 1946) stressed that diverticula occurred under the age of thirty having seen six patients with them while in their twenties and one at the age of twelve; he believed that statistics based on autopsies and barium enemas were misleading as they only took into account patients who were selected by age or by symptoms. In particular, his views were coloured by the fact that five out of seventeen cases of caecal diverticulitis were under the age of thirty, but it should be remembered that caecal diverticula may have a different aetiology; the common form of the condition is undoubtedly a disease that becomes common in middle age. Similarly, the perforated diverticula at the splenic flexure which led to the death of a baby only eighteen hours old (Arnheim, 1940) cannot be considered to be typical of diverticular disease.

Schlotthauer (1946) reported the presence of diverticula in each of seven white brothers and concluded that some congenital factor was operating, but his testimony is also unconvincing. The disease is so common in the Western nations that coincidence alone could account for the presence of diverticula in every member of an even larger family.

While it would be unwise to deny the possible occurrence of diverticula in children, it is fair to say that they must be extremely rare. However, young people in the fourth and even third decade of life are now being found with the disease, so that it must no longer be regarded as only affecting those of over forty years of age (Eusebio and Eisenberg, 1973). This change suggests that the factors which cause this acquired disease are operating more and more effectively and that diverticulitis in young patients will become a greater problem in the future.

Chapter 6

Factors that have been Considered Responsible for Diverticulosis

INTRODUCTION

The cause of diverticulosis could not be investigated until apparatus capable of recording the pressures in the diseased colon continuously was designed. Such apparatus was not available until quite recently and so it was not until 1961 that these pressures were measured accurately. Hence, it is not surprising that there has been much speculation as to the aetiology and as to the pathogenesis of the disease over the years. In this chapter the little that was known about the causation of the disease up to 1961 is discussed together with the many theories that have found their way into the literature.

Colonic diverticula are false diverticula and consist of herniations of the colonic mucosa membrane through the colonic wall. As herniation implies the existence of a propelling or pulsion force, with or without an initial defect in the integument, the causation of diverticula is a subject that has invited much speculation. Several generations of medical writers have debated the issue, some of them favouring the view that diverticula may be caused by high pressures in the bowel while others have emphasized the importance of weakness of the bowel wall. Some have thought that this weakness was congenital and some have sought to show that it was acquired. The anatomy of the normal and diseased colon and the radiological appearances of the condition had all been described in detail but, before 1961, the pressures in the living human colon remained unknown.

Before these pressures were measured accurately, some workers were forced to infer the presence of high intra-colonic pressure by interpreting the symptoms of constipation and of flatulence as evidence of intestinal distension. Others have blamed straining at stool, some unrecognized form of intestinal obstruction or some ill-defined 'spasm' of the colon for raising the intraluminal pressures and so initiating the extrusion of the colonic mucosa. The theories that have been advanced will be considered under two headings, namely those postulating some weakness of the colonic wall and those blaming increased intra-colonic pressures. The role of factors of a general nature such as age, sex, race and diet are discussed elsewhere in this book. It should be remembered that some of the theories which will be discussed have been discarded or are no longer fashionable. Finally, and most important of all, it must be stressed that any explanation of the pathogenesis of diverticula must account for an apparent paradox, namely, that the colon in producing diverticula must, at the same time, be strong enough to generate pressures which its muscle coat is too weak to withstand.

(1) THEORIES POSTULATING WEAKNESS OF THE COLONIC WALL

(a) OBESITY

Professor J. B. S. Jackson of Boston informed Gross (1845) that diverticula were usually found in the colons of old and corpulent people. Since then, others have suggested that fatty infiltration of the colon caused diverticulosis. Klebs (1869) believed that fat collected around the colon's blood vessels and further increased the gap which they made in the muscle coat; he also thought that fat-laden mesenteric vessels caused traction diverticula in the small gut. Edel (1894) reviewed the possible causes of diverticula and pointed out that they were found just as frequently in thin and wasted patients as they were in those that were overweight. Hanseman (1896) reported diverticula in a man of 85 who had always been lean while Dunn and Woolley (1911) failed to understand how fat deposited beneath the colonic serosa could affect the strength of the muscularis propria. Telling and Gruner (1917) argued that both fatty degeneration and cachexia could weaken the tissues of the colonic wall.

Clinically, no significant preponderance of fat subjects with the disease was observed by Spriggs and Marxer (1927), by Mayo (1930), by Oshner and Bargen (1936) or by Morton (1946). Accordingly, obesity has been discarded as an aetiological factor in the genesis of the disease (Horner, 1958). However, it should be remembered that both diverticular disease and obesity are common in communities who eat refined carbohydrates in quantity. Consequently, both conditions may have common causative factors (Cleave, Campbell and Painter, 1969).

(b) THE ROLE OF THE BLOOD VESSELS

The segmental vessels that serve the colon penetrate the muscularis propria in an orderly arrangement (Griffiths, 1956). The arteries give off large lateral branches that pass through the circular muscle between the taenia and, consequently, have become smaller by the time they reach the anti-mesocolic periphery of the colon. Hence, in the early stages of the disease, diverticula are seen less often between the anti-mesocolic taenia (Watt and Marcus, 1964) and are usually found at regular intervals in two rows on each side of the colon (Haberschon, 1857; Slack, 1962 and 1967). This orderly arrangement is less obvious in advanced specimens of the disease because diverticula may coalesce or burrow intramurally (Cohen, Cunningham and Snierson, 1957) a process that was observed in rats by Carlson and Hoelzel (1949).

Graser (1899) thought that venous distension in the aged suffering from dropsy might enlarge the defect around the blood vessels but Sudsuki (1900) showed that this theory was untenable in most cases. The blood vessels bear the same relationship to diverticula as does the spermatic cord to an inguinal hernia. The anatomical arrangement of these vessels is common to normal colons as well as to those which are diseased, regardless of race or ethnic origin and so, while it may be admitted freely that diverticula usually follow the course of the blood vessels, it must never be claimed that the structure of the colon is in itself responsible for the mucosal herniation. The vessels only determine the usual site of diverticula but do not cause diverticulosis.

(c) THE ANATOMY OF THE COLON'S MUSCLE COAT

The circular muscle of the colon forms a complete tube but the longitudinal muscle is gathered into three bands, the *taenia coli*, one of which is usually situated at the mesocolic border (Fig. 3). Thus, the colonic wall is congenitally thinner between the taenia and it is here that it is further weakened by the tunnel which contains the segmental blood vessels. Diverticula usually appear first between the taenia on each side of the colon. Thus, their most usual site of occurrence is selected to a great extent by the anatomy of the large bowel which differs from that of the rest of the intestine in that its outer longitudinal coat is incomplete. By contrast, the rectum, which is enclosed in two continuous sheets of muscle, is seldom the site of diverticular disease despite its having to cope with contents of the same viscosity as does the sigmoid which is the commonest site of the disease.

(d) THE ROLE OF THE APPENDICES EPIPLOICA

Klebs (1869) and Bland-Sutton (1903) thought that traction of fat-laden appendices epiploica weakened the bowel wall but, in fact, it is the anatomical relationship between the appendices epiploica, the taenia coli and the blood vessels which is responsible for diverticula being found in the appendices. This can be seen from the classical diagram of Hamilton Drummond (Fig. 3). Diverticula follow the blood vessels and track into the fat of the appendices so that they are difficult to see from the serosal surface even when their presence can be detected by palpating their contained faecoliths. This relationship explains why the diagnosis of 'torsion of an appendix epiploica' was fashionable before the existence of diverticulosis was recognized.

(e) FACTORS WHICH MIGHT WEAKEN THE WALL OF THE COLON

Some authors have assumed, in the author's opinion correctly, that almost every colon is normal at birth. Therefore, they have attributed the appearance of diverticula to an acquired fault in the colonic wall. Fatty atrophy, old age and some undefined 'primary muscle atrophy' have been blamed for diverticulosis (Edel, 1894; Beer, 1904; David, 1933). Areas of rarefaction in the muscle coat were reported by Lockhart-Mummery (1930) and Conway and Hitzrot (1931), but it was the work of Harold Edwards (1934a and b) which clearly showed that, in the 'prediverticular stage', the circular muscle is thrown into ridges between which the muscle is very thin and the blood vessels and mucosa are in close approximation and that the scene is set for the herniation of the mucosa.

However, these findings do not provide evidence of a primary weakness of the muscle coat as the abnormalities described might well represent the response of a previously normal bowel to abnormal intracolonic pressures.

It has also been suggested that bacterial action damaged the colon, the sigmoid being most affected as it is the point where faeces are delayed (Spriggs and Marxer, 1925) but this has not been substantiated. David (1933) took pains to remark on the absence of histological evidence of inflammation around diverticula. Henderson (1944) believed that inflammation preceded diverticulosis. His view was based on his radiological experience. He also reported the appearance of diverticulosis just below a colonic neoplasm which had disappeared when barium enemas were given subsequent to resection of the growth. He explained this phenomenon by postulating that the tumour had devitalized the colonic wall; it could be accounted for equally well by the fact that diverticula are reducible in the early stages of their development.

The colon, like the rest of the body, must be affected by the ageing process. Morton (1946) noticed how arterio-sclerosis and heart disease were common in patients with diverticulitis as did Painter, Almeida and Colebourne (1972). Chapman (1934) thought that disease of the mesenteric artery might lessen the elasticity of the submucosa and lead to diverticula of the small bowel; loss of this elasticity has been blamed for diverticula in Marfan's syndrome (Mielke, Beiken and Gross, 1965). The idea that arterial insufficiency may affect the colon is attractive but Griffiths (1956) showed that the marginal artery provides the sigmoid with an adequate blood supply even when the inferior mesenteric artery is occluded and doubted whether anything less than gross arterio-sclerosis could cause circulatory deficiency in the sigmoid colon.

Hughes (1969), basing his remarks on a careful post-mortem study, concluded that, although the incidence of aortic atheroma and diverticulosis increased with age, this was more the result of ageing than of any connection between the two conditions. Cleave, Campbell and Painter (1969) believe that both diseases occur in populations who eat refined carbohydrates and thus it could be expected that they should be found together frequently. Haemorrhage from diverticula has only attracted attention in the last twenty years (Fraenkel, 1954; Noer, 1955) and has become more prevalent recently and this suggests that arterial disease and diverticulosis have some aetiological factor in common (Trowell, Painter and Burkitt, 1974). An investigation into the long-term effects of arterio-sclerosis on the integument of the colon is overdue and might be very profitable; obviously vascular deficiency could devitalize the tissues of the bowel.

Similarly, a deficiency of vitamins in the diet may play a subsidiary role in diminishing the strength of the submucosa or muscle of the colon and there is little doubt that a deficiency of vitamin C and of the B group is not uncommon in Britain today especially in the aged (Brocklehurst *et al.*, 1968; Taylor, 1973).

CONCLUSION

To sum up, it is fair to say that no evidence of an initial muscle degeneration being the primary cause of diverticulosis has ever been produced. Pathological studies of the fully developed disease will obviously reveal that the bowel wall has been weakened by multiple herniations; this has been shown to be so *in vivo* by Parks and Connell (1969) but this does not prove that the colonic wall was defective from the start.

(2) THEORIES WHICH HAVE POSTULATED THAT DIVERTICULOSIS IS CAUSED BY INCREASED INTRACOLONIC PRESSURES

Whatever part structural failure of the colonic wall plays in the development of diverticulosis, the colonic mucosa must be driven from its moorings by the force of intracolonic pressure. No method of measuring this pressure accurately over long periods was available until the late nineteen-fifties (Chaudhary and Truelove, 1961) and therefore those who wrote prior to this date were forced to infer the presence of raised intra-colonic pressure from the symptoms of their patients and from radiological observations. Constipation and flatulence have been cited as evidence of colonic distension which was believed, presumably, to blow out diverticula like weak spots on a tyre. Spasm of the sigmoid is often said to exist when this part of the colon is seen to empty itself of barium during screening. It is difficult to follow the logic of some writers but their theories fall into two ill-defined groups: some have postulated the existence of a passive distending force behind a faecal column or some form of functional obstruction, and others have blamed increased activity of the colonic muscle for abnormally high intracolonic pressures.

(a) The Distension Theory of the Pathogenesis of Colonic Diverticula.

The structural similarity of diverticula of the bladder and of the colon was obvious to the earliest investigators (Cruveilhier, 1849; Gross, 1857; Bristowe, 1854; Lane, 1885) and this led them to look for 'some mechanical obstacle to the passage of the faecal matter' comparable to the bladder neck obstruction that causes vesical diverticula. Obstruction due to a growth below the site of diverticula as observed by de Mourges (Telling and Gruner, 1917) and by Hamilton Drummond (1917) is the exception rather than the rule. Consequently, it was necessary to postulate some other cause of colonic obstruction. Constipation appeared to be the obvious culprit.

Cruveilhier believed that the faecal column slowed and solidified in the sigmoid and that constipation led to straining at stool which was transmitted to the sigmoid and displaced its mucous membrane. This statement was echoed by Anderson (1946) who stated that defaecation was accompanied by pressures of up to 50mm./Hg. in the rectum and Alvarez (1958) put this figure as high as 280 mm. Hg. Despite the lack of any evidence that these pressures affect the sigmoid, habitual costiveness, constipation and straining at stool have been held responsible for diverticulosis (Bristowe, 1854; Haberschon, 1857; Miles, 1920). This theory went out of fashion when later workers showed that constipation did not invariably accompany or precede the appearance of diverticula.

Edel (1894) questioned the role of constipation as this complaint was so common in the old, while Beer (1904) thought that straining, while not the primary cause, might prove too much for the weaker colonic muscle of old people. Telling (1908) reported that seventeen of his twenty-two patients were constipated but, in his later series, only 21% were constipated while 3·5% had loose stools (Telling and Gruner, 1917). As a result of this, he changed his views and concluded that flatulent distension was an important causative factor (Telling, 1920).

Later writers recorded that diverticulosis was accompanied by constipation in from 14% to 53% of patients, by diarrhoea in from 4% to 39% while the bowels are open daily in from 14% to 29% and alternating constipation and looseness is found in from 3% to 7% of patients about 25% of whom suffer from flatulence (Spriggs and Marxer, 1925; Oschner and Bargen, 1935; Willard and Bockus, 1936; Brown and Marcley, 1937; Feldman and Morrison, 1949; Horner, 1958). Constipation is found in two thirds of those suffering from diverticulitis and from 15% to 45% have diarrhoea (Judd and Pollock, 1924; Rankin and Brown, 1930; Eggers, 1941; Bacon and Shermon, 1950; Todd, 1955) while two thirds of Todd's patients complained of flatulence and nearly as many felt distended.

The variability of the bowel habit and flatulence that accompanies diverticular disease suggests that they are symptoms of a disorder of bowel function rather than the cause of the condition (Painter, 1962) and the observation of Painter, Almeida and Colebourne (1972) that the addition of cereal fibre to the diet alters the behaviour of the bowel and relieves these very symptoms appears to confirm this statement.

Somewhat crude experiments were performed to investigate the 'distension theory'. Hauseman (1896) produced small gut diverticula in the mesenteric border of dead small gut, obtained from old subjects, by inflating it with water, but the experiment failed when he used material obtained from young people. Fraser (1933–34) had similar results. Beer (1904) rightly questioned the value of these acute experiments as diverticula formation is a chronic process and living and dead bowel are known to respond to distension differently (Chlumsky, 1899).

If simple ballooning of the colon were responsible for diverticulosis, the disease would be found in cases of volvulus, Hirschsprung's or Chaga's disease. The concept that distension alone, in the presence of little or no muscular activity, causes diverticulosis fails to fit the facts if for no other reason than that it should result in diverticula being scattered equally throughout a thin walled colon whereas they are most common in the sigmoid region where the muscle is thickest.

(b) Theories which have Postulated that Diverticulosis is Caused by Abnormal Intracolonic Pressures

(i) The Role of Colonic Muscle Activity in the Genesis of Diverticula

Lane (1885) observed that diverticula are found in that part of the sigmoid which is thick and contracted, and not on loops of thin distended bowel (Fig. 2); and suggested that diverticula were caused by powerful contractions of the muscularis propria.

Edwards (1934) studied sections taken from parts of the colonic wall which were thickened but which did not bear diverticula. These showed changes which correspond to the 'pre-diverticular state' of Spriggs and Marxer. Edwards showed that the circular muscle varied in thickness so that hillocks of muscle, that is rings of hypertrophied circular muscle seen in cross section, were interspersed with apparently atrophic muscle which was so thinned that it hardly separated the mucosa from the serosa. This bunching of the circular muscle was seen to be more marked in the later stages of the process. Edwards clearly demonstrated blood vessels in the intervals between the thickened rings of muscle which were in close proximity to the mucosa. He believed that irregular muscular spasm was responsible for this uneven distribution of the circular coat and that the pulsion force necessary for mucosal herniation was produced by muscular contraction.

Edwards's work is of the greatest significance as his demonstration of the differing thickness of the circular muscle provides anatomical grounds on which the apparent paradox of concurrent strength and weakness of the colonic wall can be explained. If the thickened muscle contracts on to its contents, it is easy to see how the mucosa would herniate through the gap between adjacent bundles of muscle where the muscle is extremely thin or has disappeared. A similar change is to be seen in the trabeculated bladder whose contractions extrude diverticula.

Stout (1923) studied diverticula of the appendix by experimenting on the appendices of living dogs and on one human appendix immediately after its surgical removal. He cut gaps in the muscle coats while carefully leaving the submucosa intact. This trauma caused the appendicular muscle to contract so that the appendix shortened and he recorded that this always caused the submucosa and mucosa to herniate through the hole in the muscle. No such 'diverticula' appeared if this procedure was carried out after the muscularis propria had lost the ability to contract. He also inflated the appendix with fluid injected into its open end after it had contracted and extruded its mucosa. He found that if these 'diverticula bearing' appendices were distended to an extent sufficient to overcome the force of the contracting muscle, then not only did the muscle relax but also the herniated mucosa was withdrawn into the ballooned appendix. He concluded that it was 'inconceivable . . . to imagine that the force of a fluid or gas, within the lumen of the appendix, could alone be sufficient to force the . . . mucosa and submucosa through a defect in the muscularis'. He believed that the 'chief active force . . . driving the mucosa and submucosa through the weak point in the muscular wall is the contraction of the circular and longitudinal muscle coats'. He thought that previous workers had . . . completely ignored the 'tremendous energy transformations which are occurring constantly in the appendix and intestine throughout life'.

His work was repeated and improved on by Wilson (1950) using freshly removed human appendices, which were fixed and sectioned afterwards. He confirmed that these 'diverticula' never appeared unless the muscle of the appendix contracted and, if this muscle failed to contract, the mucosa was not extruded through the man-made gap in the muscle coat. He came to the conclusion that even if obstruction or distension of the lumen did play some part in the production of diverticula, these never occurred in the absence of muscular activity.

Seymour Barling (1926) has left an eye witness account of what were almost certainly diverticula being produced by strong contractions of the sigmoid colon. He performed a laparotomy under spinal anaesthesia on a man of 43 whose sigmoid colon had been previously examined by a barium enema and pronounced to be in the 'pre-diverticular state'. This patient had passed blood-stained mucus per rectum and no sigmoidoscopy had been carried out because of pain. Laparotomy revealed that the sigmoid had very little fat covering it and it felt thicker than normal. The peritoneum overlying it was injected and oedematous. Barling wrote:—

'At one point the bowel suddenly narrowed to half of its previous diameter; this narrowing spread up and down for three or four inches, the bowel in this area becoming the size of the index finger and quite as firm. It was so rigid that it resisted flexion like a string of large beads very tightly threaded. While the spasm lasted, many tiny saccules appeared between the longitudinal bands; these were each segments of a circle about a third of an inch or less in diameter and lay regularly like beads along the sides of the gut. In a few seconds, the spasm passed off and a nearly normal bowel remained with faint evidence of the tiny projections indicated for a few seconds by the altered blood supply at their sites owing to the tension to which the peritoneum had been subjected. The cycle of spasm repeated itself thrice during the time the abdomen was open.'

Barling realized that these tiny projections might be incipient herniations, but surprisingly dismissed this possibility on the grounds that they were too regular in size and position. Nevertheless, his dramatic account, together with the experimental work of Stout and Wilson, leaves little doubt that it is not passive distension, but contraction of the colon that causes diverticulosis.

(ii) Possible Causes of Abnormal Activity of the Colonic Muscle

Spasm of the colon frequently accompanied the disease according to Judd and Pollock (1924) and Le Royer and White (1948) claimed that 'spastic constipation or diarrhoea' often preceded diverticulitis. Feldman and Morrison (1949) diagnosed the presence of an 'irritable spastic colon' in two thirds of their patients and Bevan (1961) believed that spasm was followed by diverticulosis. However, Edwards (1954) failed to establish on clinical grounds any causal relationship between spastic colon and the disease despite his previously held belief that spasticity was an important factor. Recently, Parks and Connell (1972) studied the motility and pressure patterns of the human colon and concluded that there was only a tenuous connection between the Irritable Colon Syndrome and diverticular disease.

The word 'spasm' has been used loosely and should not be accepted without reservation, as the criteria by which irritability and spasm of the colon are diagnosed are ill-defined. A radiologist's report of 'spasm' often means that the sigmoid appeared functionally narrowed with its lumen almost closed or that it was unwilling to admit or to retain barium. It must not be assumed that such a sigmoid harbours high pressure, however tempting this assumption may be, unless the intracolonic pressure has been measured.

Others have suggested that the colon acts abnormally following the prolonged use of purgatives (Spriggs and Marxer, 1925) because of disorders of its autonomic nerve supply (Mayo, 1930) or neuro-muscular inco-ordination (Wolf, 1931) while Willard and Bockus (1936) considered the possibility of an exaggerated 'gastro-colic reflex' altering the motility of the colon.

Lloyd-Davies (1953) suggested that a psychosomatic factor

might initiate colonic activity leading to high pressure and emotion has been shown to alter colonic motility as measured by balloons (Almy, Kern and Tulin, 1949; Almy, Hinkle, Berle and Kern, 1949; Almy, Abbott and Hinkle, 1950).

Chaudhury and Truelove (1961), using open-ended tubes, showed that emotion affects the intracolonic pressures profoundly and Painter (1962) recorded pressure waves of 40 mm./Hg in amptitude in the sigmoid colon which could be induced merely by discussing a topic that was distasteful to the patient being studied (Fig. 44).

It is tempting to suggest that other colonic disorders which are common in young people might lead on to diverticulosis in later life but, so far, no evidence of any such connection has been produced.

(iii) The Localization of Diverticulosis

The sigmoid colon is the site of election of diverticulosis. Here the contraction of the taenia and circular muscle throw the mucosa into folds like a concertina (Keith, 1910). These may narrow the colon to such an extent that the exaggerated inter-haustral folds resemble interdigitating valves (Lloyd-Davies, 1953). These structural appearances are often very localized so that there is an abrupt transition between the affected segments and the more normal proximal colon (Fig. 3). Bevan (1961) believes that the lower sigmoid forms a type of sphincter which relaxes prior to defaecation, a view that has been elaborated by Painter (1967). If the sigmoid has a special function, its physio-logical role might have some bearing on the site of election of diverticular disease.

(3) Summary of what was known about the Causation of Diverticular Disease in 1961.

Before 1961, no systematic study of the pressures in the human colon in health and in diverticulosis had been made be-cause no means of measuring these pressures accurately over long periods were available. Consequently, despite all the clinical, radiological and anatomical investigations which had been made, only the following facts were known about diverti-culosis in 1961.

(1) The disease is acquired and appears in the second half of life with increasing frequency as age advances;

(2) The sigmoid colon is almost always affected and is usually the first site at which the disease appears;

(3) Diet plays some part in the aetiology of diverticula in rats and probably influences the development of the disease in human beings.

All other theories that had been put forward rested on the deduction, made from first principles, namely that the mucosal herniation results from an inherent weakness in the muscularis propria, abnormally high intracolonic pressure or a mixture of these two factors. Fortunately, apparatus capable of recording the intracolonic pressures became available and the role of these pressures in the pathogenesis of diverticulosis was recognized. This will be described in the following chapters.

Chapter 7

The Pressures in the Human Colon in Health and in Diverticulosis

The many theories as to the cause of diverticulosis which have been put forward have been discussed in Chapter 6. The colonic wall and its musculature had been studied extensively but the pressures in the colon remained unknown for the simple reason that no apparatus capable of measuring these pressures accurately was available. The modern view of the pathogenesis of diverticular disease depended on the use of such apparatus and this was first used to study the pressures in the human colon in diverticulosis in 1961. Almost no experimental work had been done as to the cause of diverticulosis before this date and the little that was known about colonic motility was derived from techniques which made use of balloons inserted into the colons of animals and man. Unfortunately, studies that make use of balloons inserted into the gut do not record the intraluminal pressure but merely register changes in pressure within each balloon as it is compressed or distorted by the gut wall (Brody and Quigley, 1951; Painter, 1967), (Fig. 25). By contrast, open-ended water-filled polythene tubes inserted into the lumen of the bowel record accurately the pressure in the immediate vicinity of their tips and the use of such tubes coupled with cine-radiography led to the recognition of the mechanism responsible for the herniation of the colonic mucosa (Painter, 1962 and 1964; Arfwidsson, 1964; Painter and Truelove, 1964a, b, c and d).

(1) MODERN RESEARCH

Sven Arfwidsson (1964) of Gothenburg recorded the intra-sigmoid pressures with two open-ended, fluid-filled tubes while the patient was at rest and then for a further period following a meal. Then Neostigmine was given to the patient and the recording was continued to see the effect of this drug on the

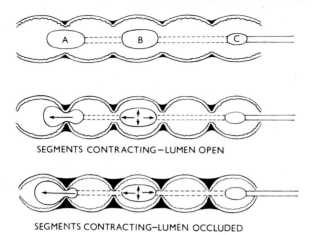

SEGMENTS CONTRACTING – LUMEN OPEN

SEGMENTS CONTRACTING – LUMEN OCCLUDED

FIG. 25. Diagram to show why balloons do not record pressure in the colon. Balloons A and B are of the same size, but it is obvious from the diagrams that they may be distorted in a different fashion depending on their relationship to the contraction rings in the bowel. This is most obvious in the lowest longitudinal section of gut when balloon A is distorted entirely differently from balloon B. Obviously, a small balloon (C) would be less liable to this distortion and, the smaller the balloon, the less would it be buffeted by contraction rings. However, the membrane of balloon C would still vary in consistency and, on occasions, the balloon would still act as a foreign body. An open-ended, fluid-filled tube does not have the same disadvantages. (From Painter, 1967.)

intracolonic pressures. He investigated 20 healthy subjects and 20 patients with diverticulosis. He found that more pressure was generated by the diseased colon than by the healthy colon while at rest. This difference was not statistically significant when the average value for each group was calculated and there was an overlap in many cases. However, after feeding, the colon that was beset with diverticula produced many more waves of pressure greater than 30 cm. of H_2O than did the normal colon postprandially. After food, the diseased colon frequently produced many more waves of high pressure (Fig. 45).

He reported that Neostigmine (0·5 mg.) given intravenously caused a striking increase in the number of waves of high pressure for a period of ten minutes, both in the normal and in the diseased colon when compared with the number recorded at rest or postprandially. Arfwidsson concluded that this different response of the diseased colon was of aetiological significance. He proceeded to demonstrate similar pressure patterns at rest, after food and after neostigmine in colons that did not bear diverticula but which radiologically showed the corrugated or 'saw toothed' appearance that is seen in diverticulosis. This corresponds to the 'pre-diverticular stage' of earlier writers and he considered that these findings showed that some change in the colonic muscle and in its behaviour preceded the appearance of diverticula. In other words, diverticula were not the primary abnormality in diverticular disease.

In 1961, Painter and Truelove carried out similar studies using the method of Chaudhary and Truelove (1961). Their work will now be described in some detail. They inserted three water-filled open-ended polythene tubes into the sigmoid colon through a sigmoidoscope, which was then withdrawn, leaving the tubes *in situ*. The tubes were tied together so that their tips were 7·5 cm. apart and each tip was bound with a metal cuff to permit radiological visualization of the point of recording. The position of the tubes was ascertained radiologically after filling the tube furthest up the colon with a fine suspension of barium (hypaque). When a patient with diverticulosis was studied, this x-ray was compared with the barium enema films in order to determine which of the recording tips was situated in segments of the colon that bore diverticula.

The polythene tubes were coupled to three Shillingford-Muller transducers whose signals were fed into a Cambridge three-channel pressure recorder which gave a direct written record of the pressure changes registered by each tube. The Cambridge recorder had a stable base-line which made it possible to record the intraluminal pressures accurately for several hours without the need for recalibration of the instrument. It yielded permanent records which could be studied at leisure (Painter and Truelove, 1964a). Prior to their work and that of Arfwidsson, no systematic observations had been made and the pressures in the human colon in health and in diverticulosis were unknown (Thompson, 1959). Painter and Truelove investigated a total of 98 volunteers. The pattern of pressures at rest were recorded for one hour and then a drug was given and the 'post-drug pattern of pressures' was recorded for a further hour. Sometimes another drug was then given and the recording was continued. The Cambridge recorder was set to register a maximum of 90 mm./Hg. At times simultaneous cineradiographic films were exposed at the rate of one frame per second. The exposure of each frame was automatically recorded on the pressure tracing so that the configuration of the colon around the recording tip could be correlated with the intraluminal pressure recorded by that tip. When cine-films were exposed, only two channels were available for pressure recording as the third was adapted to record the exposure of each frame of film.

The pressure tracings thus obtained were analysed in a number of ways. The tube furthest up the colon was called, 'Lead 1', the middle tube was labelled 'Lead 2' and the tube whose tip was nearest to the anus was labelled 'Lead 3'. Data obtained from recording leads whose tip was judged to be below the recto-sigmoid junction was excluded from their studies. Leads whose tips were situated in segments of the colon that bore diverticula were said to be *'related to diverticula'*, while leads whose tips recorded from apparently normal segments of colon in subjects with diverticulosis were designated leads *'not related to diverticula'*. The reason for this subdivision will become apparent later.

(2) RESTING PRESSURE PATTERNS IN THE NORMAL SIGMOID COLON

The patterns of pressure in 'normal' subjects and in patients with diverticulosis were compared. Normal subjects had no history of bowel dysfunction and their barium studies were normal. These control subjects were on average younger than those with diverticulosis and might well develop diverticulosis in later life but in a population prone to the disease this limitation was accepted. Thirty-three observations were made on 32 normal subjects yielding a total of 66 tracings for analysis and 29 observations were made on 28 patients with diverticulosis giving 20 tracings from leads related to diverticula and 31 from leads not related to diverticula (Table 1). For later study, Painter and Truelove found that, under resting conditions, the normal human sigmoid colon harbours a basal pressure that is within a few millimeters of mercury of the atmospheric pressure. On this basal pressure small waves of positive pressure are superimposed at irregular intervals. Usually they occur singly but occasionally in series (Fig. 26). The majority of waves last between 10 and 30 seconds and rise to a height of less than 10 mm./Hg and, occasionally, waves exceeding 60 mm./Hg were

TABLE 1

NUMBER OF SUBJECTS STUDIED, OBSERVATIONS MADE, AND LEADS
FROM WHICH PRESSURE TRACINGS WERE OBTAINED

	Number of Subjects	Number of Observations	Number of Leads Analysed
Normal subjects	32	33	66
Patients with diverticulosis	28	29	20 (related to diverticula) 31 (not related to diverticula)

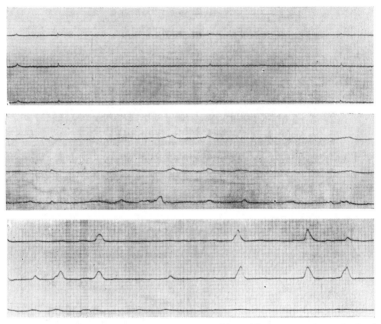

FIG. 26. Resting pressure patterns in the normal sigmoid colon. Tracings obtained from normal sigmoid colons; only lead 3 in the top tracing was not located above the rectosigmoid junction. Each tracing represents six minutes of recording time; this scale has been adhered to throughout this book unless otherwise stated. The variation in the number and dimensions of the pressure waves occurring in the sigmoid can be seen. The highest wave in the top tracing represents 30 mm. Hg pressure, while in the lowest tracing the intraluminal pressure hardly altered except for the small changes caused by respiration. (Reproduced from Painter and Truelove, 1964a.)

recorded (Table 2). Sometimes waves of pressure were recorded at all three levels in the gut while at other times one or more of the tracings remained at the basal level. When waves of pressure were recorded they occurred independently of each other and it was extremely rare to find waves of the same dimension occurring simultaneously at each level of the bowel. When waves were

TABLE 2

NUMBER OF WAVES BY AMPLITUDE OF WAVE IN SIGMOID COLON[1]

Amplitude of Waves (mm. Hg)	Normal	Resting Values Diverticulosis	
		Leads not Related to Diverticula	Leads Related to Diverticula
1–9	34·7	35·2	25·2
10–19	2·3	3·8	4·4
20–29	0·9	0·6	0·6
30–39	0·3	0·2	0·5
40–49	0·3	0·2	0·3
50–59	0·3	0·1	0·3
60 +	0·02	0·1	0·05
Total	38·6	40·2	31·3

[1] Mean values per lead per 60 minutes' recording time.

recorded simultaneously at more than one level their form was usually different. No evidence of the anal-ward progression of a pocket of high pressure was obtained except when wind was passed (Fig. 27). No attempt was made to classify these waves into the Types I, II and III of earlier writers who used balloons. The great variation in the number of pressure waves produced in normal subjects that had been reported by Chaudhary and

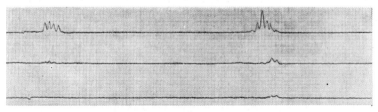

FIG. 27. The effect of passing flatus. All leads situated in sigmoid colon of patient with diverticulosis, leads 1 and 2 being related to diverticula. The tracing remained at the resting basal level of pressure except when flatus was passed. This 'progression' of pressure towards the anus was not seen at any other time.

Truelove (1961) was observed again and their findings were confirmed.

Painter and Truelove concluded that observations from a considerable number of control subjects were required in order to establish a yard stick against which the pressures in diverticulosis could be compared and so they made thirty-three observations. They realized that the normal sigmoid could localize pressure to the region of one recording tip although the mechanism responsible for this was not then apparent.

(3) RESTING PRESSURE PATTERNS IN THE SIGMOID COLON IN DIVERTICULOSIS

When they examined the pressure tracings obtained from diseased colons to see if they differed from the 'normal' tracings, no obvious difference was found. The size, shape, irregular occurrence and lack of any temporal relationship between a wave at one level of the sigmoid and waves at adjoining levels that had been found in the normal colon were also seen in diverticulosis (Fig. 28).

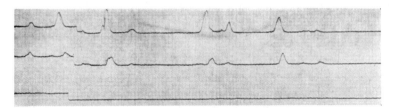

FIG. 28. Resting pressure pattern in sigmoid bearing diverticula. The sudden drop in the basal level on the left of the tracing was due to the deliberate re-selling of the recording pens. Waves of over 60 mm. Hg are shown on lead 1 but these high pressures are not recorded by lead 2 which was only 7·5 cm. distant. This shows that the colon can localize pressures. The comparison of this tracing with Fig. 27 shows the great variation in the pattern of pressures that occur in diverticular disease.

No obvious increase in the pressures in the colon were seen in tracings derived from patients with diverticulosis.

Detailed analysis of the pressure tracings confirmed this impression and this failure to detect any difference between the normal resting pattern and the pattern in diverticulosis led to a further analysis of the tracings. When it was remembered that the segments of the sigmoid that actually bear diverticula are often structurally different from the neighbouring colon, from which they may be sharply demarcated (Fig. 1), Painter and Truelove considered that this anatomical difference might be reflected in an equally abrupt change of function as regards the generation of intraluminal pressures. Consequently, tracings derived from leads whose tips were situated in segments bearing diverticula were analysed separately from those whose tips were located in apparently normal bowel in patients with diverticulosis. Thus, '*resting patterns related to diverticula*' and '*resting*

TABLE 3
NUMBER OF WAVES BY DURATION OF WAVE IN SIGMOID COLON[1]

Duration of Waves (sec.)	Resting Values		
	Normal	Diverticulosis	
		Leads not Related to Diverticula	Leads Related to Diverticula
1–9	10·7	13·1	8·3
10–19	17·7	16·9	11·9
20–29	7·3	7·3	6·6
30–39	1·73	1·48	2·4
40–49	0·5	0·94	1·2
50–59	0·4	0·39	0·8
60 +	0·3	0·13	0·15
Total	38·6	40·2	31·3

[1] Mean values per lead per 60 minutes' recording time.

patterns not related to diverticula' were studied but, once again, no obvious difference was apparent in the two types of resting patterns and quantitative analysis of the tracings, which will be described later, confirmed that this impression was correct.

(4) QUANTITATIVE ASPECTS OF PRESSURE WAVES IN SIGMOID COLON IN HEALTH AND IN DIVERTICULOSIS

Painter and Truelove measured the number of waves of pressure of differing amplitudes and different duration. The height and duration of each wave was measured, regardless of the complexity of its shape. Thus they obtained values for the mean number of waves of various dimensions per lead per 60 minutes of recording time. This method had been used by Chaudhary and Truelove (1961). When these figures were examined (see Tables 2 and 3), no significant difference in the pressures derived from the three types of segments was found. Over 80% of the waves in each group of tracings were of an amplitude less than 10 mm./Hg and, under basal conditions, no preponderance of high pressure waves were found to occur near to diverticula. When the duration of the waves was considered, it was found that 80% of the waves lasted less than 30 seconds but segments that bore diverticula did produce more waves of a duration greater than 30 seconds than did the normal segments.

Chaudhary and Truelove (1961) proposed that a 'Colonic Motility Index' could be calculated by multiplying the height of the wave against its duration. As most waves are roughly triangular in shape, the product of these two factors would yield a figure approximately double the area enclosed by the wave. This area is proportional to the work done (i.e. pressure x time) by the colon in generating these pressures. When these values were plotted (Fig. 35), it was apparent that, despite the variations of the indices in each column, the average values were almost the same. This was at variance with Arfwidsson's findings to some extent. However, when the individual variations in the pressures among patients and the limitations of the methods employed are taken into account, there is little to suggest that the pressures in the normal and diseased sigmoid colon differ significantly under basal conditions. This has since been substantiated by Attisha and Smith (1969) and by Smith and his colleagues (1969) in Edinburgh while, in Belfast, Parks (1970) inserted small balloons into the colon and came to a similar conclusion.

Thus several studies have failed to produce any convincing evidence that, under resting conditions, diverticular disease is accompanied by 'intraluminal hypertension'.

Chapter 8

The Effect of Certain Drugs and other Stimuli on the Pressures in the Human Colon

When it was found that the pressures in the normal sigmoid colon did not differ significantly, under basal conditions, from those in the diseased colon, the effect of other stimuli, including certain drugs, upon these pressures was investigated by various workers. It was found that some drugs increased the intracolonic pressures while others had the reverse effect. The clinical importance of these findings will be discussed as will be the observation of Arfwidsson (1964) and other workers that the sigmoid colon is activated after meals and that this effect is more marked in patients with diverticulosis.

(1) THE EFFECT OF MORPHINE

(a) The Effect of Morphine on the Pressures in the Normal Colon

Morphine is still the most important analgesic but its effect on the human intestinal muscle and the intraluminal pressures was not known until Painter and Truelove (1964b) measured these pressures in a manner similar to that used to record the resting pressures both in health and in diverticulosis and also after 10 mg. of Morphine Sulphate had been given either intravenously or intramuscularly. One hour's recording from each lead was analysed in the same way as were the tracings from the resting bowel. Intravenous morphine produced a sudden change in the pressure tracings derived from the normal bowel almost at once (Fig. 29). After the drug was given, several waves of high pressure occurred in quick succession. This cycle of events would continue for several minutes. These dramatic changes were usually followed by the pressure remaining at the basal level for several minutes before another series of waves was generated. The height of these waves varied from lead to lead but the base line pressure remained within a millimetre or two of the atmospheric pressure. The 'post-morphine pattern of

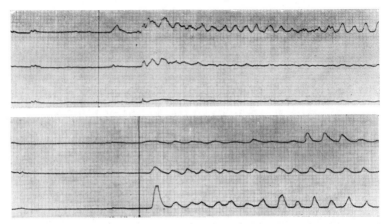

FIG. 29. The effect of an intravenous injection of morphine on the intrasigmoid pressures. The vertical line indicates the completion of the injection. The upper tracing was obtained from three leads in a normal sigmoid colon, which reacted to the injection within 16 seconds. In the lower tracing, lead 1 was related to diverticula, lead 2 was in the sigmoid below the level of diverticula, and lead 3 was at the recto-sigmoid junction. Lead 1 recorded pressures approaching 50 mm. Hg near the diverticula following morphine.

pressures' consisted of a rhythmical succession of small waves (Fig. 30). These appeared to arise independently at each level of the gut because no temporal relationship was detected which

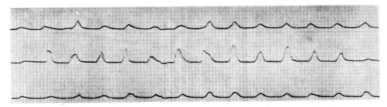

FIG. 30. Pressure pattern in normal sigmoid after morphine. All three leads were in the sigmoid colon of a woman of 48 who had been given morphine. Waves of pressure occurred rhythmically at all three levels of the sigmoid. The similarity of the form of successive waves suggests that they were produced by a similar mechanism.

suggested that these pressures proceeded towards the anus. These waves of pressure were usually less than 20 mm./Hg in amplitude. Intramuscular morphine produced similar changes after an interval of about 15 minutes. It became obvious that the normal sigmoid colon could localize pressure to one or two segments because recording tips situated only 7·5 cm. on either side of this zone of high pressure were unaffected by it (Fig. 31).

The mechanism responsible for the generation and localization of these pressures is now known to involve segmentation (Painter *et al.*, 1965).

(b) Effect of Morphine on the Pressures in Diverticulosis Coli

The 'post-morphine' patterns were divided into two groups, 'related to diverticula' and 'not related to diverticula' as had

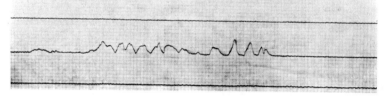

FIG. 31. Localization of pressure in normal sigmoid colon after morphine. All three leads were in a normal sigmoid colon. Lead 2 recorded pressures of up to 40 mm. Hg, but no change of pressure was registered by leads 1 and 3, whose tips were situated on either side of lead 2 at a distance of 7·5 cm. Obviously the sigmoid can localize high pressures to a short length of its lumen.

been done with the resting patterns. The apparently normal segments in patients with diverticulosis produced patterns similar to those seen in the normal colon after morphine.

However, the tracings derived from diseased segments bearing diverticula obviously differed from those already described (Fig. 32). Although the same rhythmic pattern of pressure production was seen, bouts of activity were interspersed with very high waves which sometimes exceeded 90 mm./Hg. These sometimes occurred in quick succession; up to 20 such waves have been seen to follow one another, being separated by intervals of only a few seconds. Analysis showed that, when activated by morphine, segments which bear diverticula generate higher pressures more often than do apparently normal segments in patients with diverticulosis. Furthermore, these high pressures can be localized to the immediate vicinity of one recording tip.

(c) Quantitative Aspects of the Pressures evoked by Morphine in Diverticulosis Coli

Table 4 shows the number of patients studied and Table 5 the number of waves of various heights recorded per lead per hour from the various types of segments. Morphine increased the number of pressure waves in all groups of segments. After

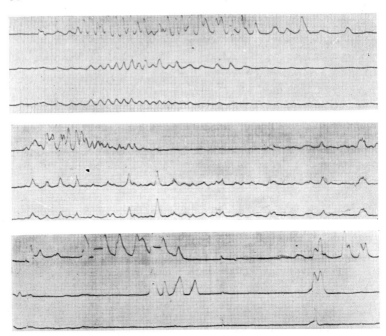

FIG. 32 . Pressure patterns in diverticulosis after morphine. In the upper tracing leads 1 and 2 were located in segments bearing diverticula. Lead 1 registered pressures of up to 60 mm. Hg. Similar high pressures occurred after morphine in segments that bore diverticula in a patient recovering from acute diverticulitis (lead 1 of middle tracing), while leads 2 and 3, which were below the level of diverticula, registered lower pressures. Leads 1 and 2 of the bottom tracing were related to diverticula and recorded very high pressures of up to 76 mm. Hg. The high pressures registered by lead 1 were not constantly recorded by lead 2, thus demonstrating the ability of the sigmoid to localize pressure.

morphine, waves of moderate height between 20 and 50 mm./Hg were doubled in frequency in the normal colon, nearly quadrupled in the 'not related' group but became ten times more frequent in segments bearing diverticula (Fig. 33). When waves of over 50 mm./Hg were considered (Fig. 34), it became apparent that such waves only occurred about once in five hours in the 'normal' segments but about once in every 24 minutes in segments that bore diverticula.

This showed that the affected segments were capable of a different response as regards the height of the waves they generated but, when the duration of these waves was studied, no differential response was found (Table 6). Calculation of the

TABLE 4
NUMBER OF SUBJECTS STUDIED, OBSERVATIONS MADE, AND LEADS
FROM WHICH PRESSURE TRACINGS WERE OBTAINED AFTER MORPHINE

	Number of Subjects	Number of Observations	Number of Leads Analysed
Normal subjects	21	21	42
Subjects with diverticulosis	25	26	19 (related to diverticula) 26 (not related to diverticula)

TABLE 5
NUMBER OF WAVES BY AMPLITUDE OF WAVE IN SIGMOID
COLON AFTER ADMINISTRATION OF MORPHINE[1]

Amplitude of Waves (mm. Hg)	Normal	Diverticulosis	
		Leads not Related to Diverticula	Leads Related to Diverticula
1–9	58·2	70·7	67·7
10–19	10·2	13·9	23·8
20–29	1·9	2·5	8·4
30–39	0·8	1·0	3·9
40–49	0·3	0·2	1·9
50–59	0·05	0·1	1·3
60+	0·0	0·2	1·3
Total	71·4	88·6	108·3

[1] Mean values per lead per 60 minutes' recording time.

TABLE 6
NUMBER OF WAVES BY DURATION OF WAVE IN SIGMOID
COLON AFTER ADMINISTRATION OF MORPHINE[1]

Duration of Waves (sec.)	Normal	Diverticulosis	
		Leads not Related to Diverticula	Leads Related to Diverticula
1–9	14·0	20·2	24·6
10–19	40·0	44·5	60·1
20–29	12·9	14·8	14·6
30–39	2·0	4·9	4·6
40–49	1·4	1·6	2·0
50–59	0·6	1·3	1·3
60+	0·5	1·3	1·1
Total	71·4	88·6	108·3

[1] Mean values per lead per 60 minutes' recording time.

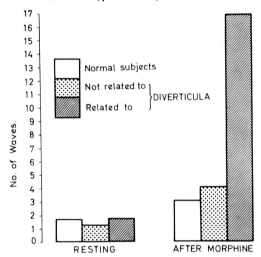

FIG. 33. Average number of waves exceeding 20 mm. Hg in height (per lead per hour) in the sigmoid colon before and after morphine.

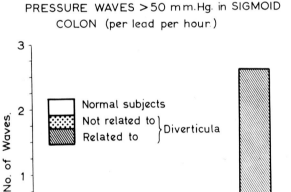

FIG. 34. Average number of waves exceeding 50 mm. Hg in height (per lead per hour) in the sigmoid colon before and after morphine.

colonic motility indices confirmed that the diseased segments produced more pressure after morphine than did the other types of segments (Fig. 35). Later, cineradiography showed that these high pressures inflated diverticula to an alarming degree. Painter and Truelove (1963) warned that the use of morphine as an analgesic in acute diverticulitis might predispose to the perforation of diverticula.

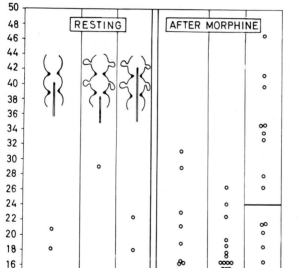

Fig. 35. Colonic motility index: resting and 'post-morphine' values. The horizontal lines represent the mean values of indices in each column.

(2) THE EFFECT OF PROSTIGMINE ON THE
INTRASIGMOID PRESSURES

Prostigmine (neostigmine methyl sulphate) was introduced in 1931 as a gastrointestinal stimulant. Its parasympatheticomimetic actions are due to its ability to inhibit cholinesterase but it may have a direct effect on autonomic ganglia. It is believed that an intact nerve supply to the gut is necessary for it to exert its full effect, which is greatest on the colon (Goodman and Gillman, 1955). Thus prostigmine enhances the effects of any impulses that activate the colon and so probably accentuates the motor activity induced by naturally occurring stimuli. Its effect on the colon was studied by Arfwidsson (1964) and by Painter and Truelove (1964c). The latter wished to see whether the drug produced an exaggerated response of the diverticula-bearing segments of the sigmoid colon similar to that which is evoked by morphine. Table 7 gives the number of subjects studied and the tracings obtained while Tables 8 and 9 present the mean values of the pressure waves of varying dimensions that were recorded in the course of one hour before and after prostigmine from the subjects studied.

TABLE 7

NUMBER OF SUBJECTS STUDIED AND LEADS FROM WHICH
PRESSURE TRACINGS WERE OBTAINED IN THE STUDY OF
NEOSTIGMINE METHYLSULPHATE (PROSTIGMINE)

	Number of Subjects *(Each Studied Once)*	*Leads in Sigmoid*
Normal subjects	12	26
Subjects with diverticulosis	12	9 (related to diverticula) 11 (not related to diverticula)

The effect of the intramuscular injection of 1 mg. of prostigmine became apparent after about 15 minutes and its effect often began to wane after one hour. The drug generally increased the number of pressure waves in the normal colon and elicited high waves of long duration more frequently.

These waves were frequently complex in shape and often consisted of several peaks whose descending strokes did not

TABLE 8

NUMBER OF WAVES BY AMPLITUDE OF WAVE IN SIGMOID COLON BEFORE AND AFTER ADMINISTRATION OF NEOSTIGMINE METHYLSULPHATE (PROSTIGMINE)[1]

Amplitude of Wave (mm. Hg)	Resting Values			Post-prostigmine Values		
	Normal	Diverticulosis		Normal	Diverticulosis	
		Not Related	Related		Not Related	Related
1–9	29·00	33·09	30·33	39·42	45·73	33·78
10–19	3·23	3·64	4·89	12·96	19·18	15·22
20–29	1·58	0·91	1·78	6·23	5·91	6·78
30–39	0·54	0·64	1·11	2·88	2·55	5·33
40–49	0·50	0·18	0·67	2·15	2·64	1·33
50–59	0·38	0·09	0·56	1·15	0·82	1·22
60+	0·19	0·09	0·11	1·12	0·45	2·46
Total	35·42	38·64	39·45	65·91	77·28	66·12

[1] Mean values per lead per 60 minutes' recording time.

return to the base line (Fig. 36). Such waves differed from those seen at rest or after morphine. Prostigmine did not evoke rhythmically occurring groups of waves to the same extent as did morphine.

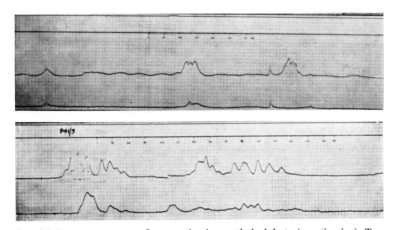

Fig. 36. Pressure patterns after neostigmine methylsulphate (prostigmine). Two tracings, each representing three minutes of recording time, in which the top pressure-recording channel had been modified to record the exposure of a simultaneously-exposed cineradiographic film. The upper tracing shows pressure waves recorded from a normal sigmoid colon after prostigmine. The lower tracing was obtained from two leads in the sigmoid colon of a man of 46 with diverticulosis who had been given prostigmine. Such multi-peaked and complex waves were seen after prostigmine both in health and in diverticulosis.

When the pressure tracings derived from patients with diverticulosis after prostigmine were observed, there did not appear to be any obvious difference between tracings derived from segments bearing diverticula and tracings belonging to leads that were recording from apparently unaffected segments in patients with diverticulosis. After prostigmine waves of all sizes were increased in number, but their form differed little from those seen after prostigmine in normal patients. Quantitative analysis showed that waves of less than 10 mg. Hg were increased by about one third after prostigmine except in the diseased segments. Waves of over 20 mg. Hg were recorded at least four times as often except from leads not related to diverticula where they were seven times more frequent. The reason for these variations is not known.

Painter and Truelove found that the segments that bore

diverticula produced the greatest number of waves of over 50 mm. Hg in amplitude but that the differential response of these segments was not as marked as that which is seen after morphine, (Fig 37). However, when the duration of waves was considered, it was found that prostigmine caused the diseased segments to generate pressures of longer duration than did the other segments and that this difference was more marked than after morphine (Table 9). Obviously, the two drugs affect the colon differently.

When the Colonic Motility Index was calculated (Fig. 38) it became apparent that when both amplitude and duration of waves was taken into consideration, the segments that bore diverticula produced more pressure after prostigmine than did the normal colon or the apparently normal segments in the diseased sigmoid. This observation was confirmed by Attisha and Smith (1969) except in two patients whose colon had been grossly affected by the disease and had become fibrosed. Recurrent inflammation may convert the colon into a hypoactive fibrous tube which can no longer generate pressure (Smith *et al.*, 1969).

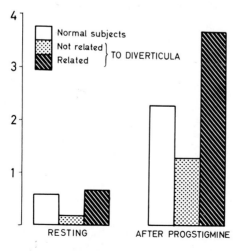

PRESSURE WAVES > 50mm. Hg. in Sigmoid colon (per lead, per hour.)

Normal subjects
Not related ⎫
Related ⎬ TO DIVERTICULA

RESTING   AFTER PROGSTIGMINE

Fig. 37. Average number of waves exceeding 50 mm. Hg in height (per lead per hour) in the sigmoid before and after neostigmine methylsulphate (prostigmine).

TABLE 9

NUMBER OF WAVES BY DURATION OF WAVE IN SIGMOID COLON BEFORE AND AFTER
ADMINISTRATION OF NEOSTIGMINE METHYLSULPHATE (PROSTIGMINE)[1]

Duration of Wave (mm. Hg)	Resting Values			Post-prostigmine Values		
	Normal	Diverticulosis		Normal	Diverticulosis	
		Not Related	Related		Not Related	Related
1–9	8·42	13·75	12·33	10·50	20·00	10·11
10–19	18·08	16·27	16·67	34·23	37·73	22·11
20–29	6·15	5·91	6·44	13·73	12·73	14·33
30–39	1·58	1·55	1·89	3·53	3·64	7·78
40–49	0·65	0·82	1·22	1·92	1·55	4·56
50–59	0·23	0·18	0·56	0·96	0·73	3·11
60 +	0·31	0·18	0·33	1·23	0·91	4·11
Total	35·42	38·64	39·44	65·92	77·29	66·11

[1] Mean values per lead per 60 minutes' recording time.

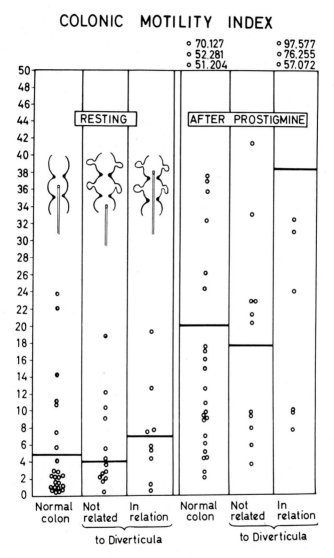

FIG. 38. Colonic motility index: resting and post-prostigmine values. The horizontal lines represent the mean values of the indices in each column.

Such a colon was studied by cineradiography by Painter (1962). This was so rigid that the necks of some diverticula could not alter in size and remained wide open, presumably due to scarring of the surrounding muscle fibres, even when high pressures were generated by the neighbouring colon in response to the administration of morphine. Thus diverticula arising from a rigid fibrous part of the sigmoid may be exposed to the full force of any intracolonic pressures that are produced by adjacent segments of the colon which still have the power to contract spontaneously or in response to drugs.

The use of neostigmine by anaesthetists to reverse the action of muscle relaxants appears to raise the pressures in the colon and the ileum sufficiently to disrupt ileo-rectal anastomoses (Bell and Lewis, 1968) and this effect is not blocked completely by the simultaneous administration of atropine (Wilkins, Hardcastle, Mann and Kaufman, 1970). In view of these observations, the wisdom of using prostigmine or morphine during or following operations involving the large bowel must be questioned.

(3) THE EFFECT OF MEPERIDINE HYDRO-CHLORIDE (PETHIDINE, DEMEROL)

Painter and Truelove (1963 and 1964) concluded that morphine might be dangerous as an analgesic in the treatment of acute diverticulitis because it raised the intracolonic pressures and might predispose to perforation. Hence, they studied the effect of Pethidine (Demerol) on these pressures, as this drug had been said to relax smooth muscle and so it was hoped that it would not raise the intracolonic pressures. This was found to be the case. They gave 100 milligrams of meperidine hydrochloride intramuscularly to six normal subjects and to five patients with diverticulosis and recorded the 'post-drug pressure patterns' for one hour. Pressure tracings from 15 leads whose tips were situated in normal segments were then compared with seven tracings derived from diverticula-bearing segments and with three tracings derived from apparently normal segments in patients with diverticular disease. The resting patterns of pressure in the normal and in the diseased colon were essentially similar to those which have been already described.

Pethidine diminished the frequency of waves of all sizes both in health and in diverticulosis. On average, the drug became effective about 12 minutes after its intramuscular injection but its effect was not dramatic. The most noticeable effect of the 'post-pethidine' pattern was a prolongation of the periods between the production of pressure waves. Frequently, the intrasigmoid pressure remained at the basal level for several minutes on end and this was always within a few mm./Hg of the atmospheric pressure (Fig. 39).

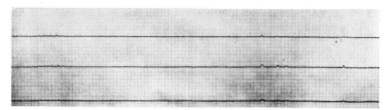

FIG. 39. Effect of pethidine on pressure patterns in sigmoid colon. All three leads were in a normal sigmoid colon; the only changes of pressure recorded in six minutes were due to respiration. After pethidine, the pressure tracing frequently remained flat for several minutes.

When the dimensions and the number of waves were examined quantitatively, it became apparent that waves of all amplitudes were diminished in frequency after pethidine (Table 10).

In contrast to morphine, pethidine reduced and almost abolished the production of waves of high pressure both in healthy and in diverticula-bearing segments. This is shown graphically in Fig. 40. Only one wave greater than 50 mm./Hg was recorded after pethidine during the 11 hours that the intrasigmoid pressures were measured in healthy control subjects and in patients with diverticulosis. No remarkable effect of the drug on the duration of the waves was observed (Table 11).

Calculation of the Colonic Motility Index confirmed that pethidine was found to lower the total pressure generated by both the healthy and the diseased colon (Fig. 41). Painter and Truelove (1964d) concluded that pethidine (demerol) is the drug of choice for the relief of pain in the treatment of acute diverticulitis because it lowers the intraluminal pressures and hence does not predispose to the perforation of inflamed diverticula as does morphine.

TABLE 10
NUMBER OF WAVES BY AMPLITUDE OF WAVE IN SIGMOID COLON BEFORE AND AFTER THE ADMINISTRATION OF PETHIDINE[1]

Amplitude of Wave (mm. Hg)	Resting Values			Post-pethidine Values		
	Normal	Diverticulosis		Normal	Diverticulosis	
		Not Related	Related		Not Related	Related
1–9	26·0	31·00	61·71	14·47	7·67	22·29
10–19	1·73	6·00	5·00	1·80	1·33	0·86
20–29	0·80	1·33	1·00	0·47	0·00	0·29
30–39	0·33	0·33	0·29	0·13	0·00	0·14
40–49	0·33	0·00	0·14	0·06	0·00	0·00
50–59	0·06	0·00	0·00	0·00	0·00	0·00
60+	0·00	0·00	0·00	0·00	0·00	0·00
Total	29·25	38·66	68·14	16·93	9·00	23·58

[1] Mean values per lead per 60 minutes' recording time.

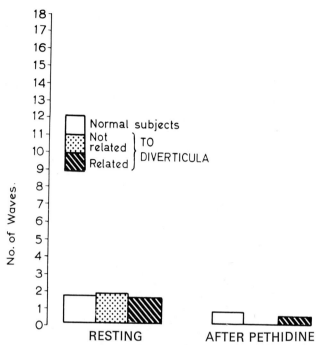

PRESSURE WAVES > 20 mm. Hg. in SIGMOID COLON (per lead per hour.)

Fig. 40. Average number of waves exceeding 20 mm. Hg in height (per lead per hour) in sigmoid colon before and after pethidine.

(4) THE EFFECT OF PROPANTHELINE BROMIDE (PROBANTHINE)

Probanthine (propantheline bromide) relaxes the colon. Lumsden and Truelove (1959) used this drug as an adjunct to barium enema examinations to aid in the differentiation of colonic lesions. The drug paralyses the bowel muscle so that it becomes an inert tube with a greatly increased diameter with indistinct haustral markings. Painter and Truelove (1964d) administered either 15 mg. or 30 mg. of probanthine intravenously to six healthy subjects and to six patients with diverticulosis all of whom had received morphine in the previous hour.

The effect of intravenous probanthine was dramatic. The drug stopped the production of pressure waves usually within 30

TABLE 11

NUMBER OF WAVES BY DURATION OF WAVE IN SIGMOID COLON BEFORE AND AFTER
THE ADMINISTRATION OF PETHIDINE[1]

Duration of Wave (sec.)	Resting Values				Post-pethidine Values			
	Normal	Diverticulosis			Normal	Diverticulosis		
		Not Related	Related			Not Related	Related	
1–9	11·07	8·33	23·57		6·47	5·67	7·14	
10–19	13·87	23·00	27·14		6·07	2·00	10·29	
20–29	2·87	5·33	11·71		2·47	0·67	4·71	
30–39	0·93	1·00	3·29		1·00	0·33	1·00	
40–49	0·27	0·66	1·29		0·47	0·00	0·43	
50–59	0·13	0·33	1·00		0·06	0·00	0·00	
60+	0·13	0·00	0·14		0·40	0·33	0·00	
Total	29·27	28·67	68·14		16·94	9·00	23·57	

[1] Mean values per lead per 60 minutes' recording time.

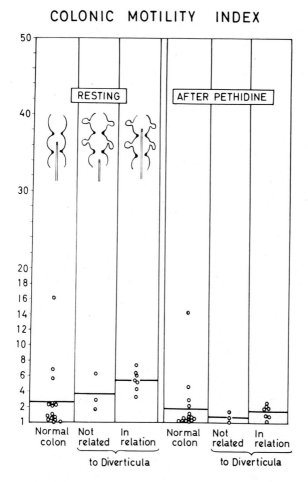

FIG. 41. Colonic motility index: resting and post-pethidine values.

seconds and always within one minute of its injection. The pressure waves that followed the use of morphine disappeared almost immediately and the intrasigmoid pressure then remained within 4 mm./Hg of atmospheric pressure. Even in patients who had only recently suffered from acute diverticulitis, probanthine completely abolished the high pressures that morphine had evoked (Fig. 42). Probanthine has also been shown to abolish the pressures that followed the administration of prostigmine.

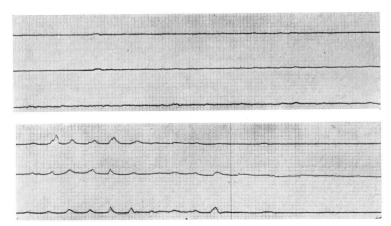

Fɪɢ. 42. Effect of propantheline bromide (probanthine) on the pressures that follow the use of morphine. Intravenous probanthine almost immediately stopped the generation of pressure waves that had followed the administration of morphine to a healthy subject. The vertical line in the upper tracing indicates the completion of the injection. The pressure tracing remained flat for the remainder of the experiment which lasted a further thirty minutes. Probanthine has the same effect in diverticulosis, and completely suppressed the production of high pressures that morphine had revoked in a patient recovering from diverticulosis (lower tracing). The effect of morphine on the intra-sigmoid pressures in the patient can be seen in the middle tracing of Figure 32 in this chapter.

(5) THE EFFECT OF EATING

The observation that the segments of the colon which are beset with diverticula respond differently when activated by morphine and prostigmine helped to elucidate the pathogenesis of the disease but, obviously, these man-made stimuli do not affect the colon in everyday life. Consequently, the work of Arfwidsson (1964) in recording the effect of a naturally occurring stimulus, namely eating, on the intrasigmoid pressures is of the greatest importance, (Fig. 43).

After he had studied the resting pressures, he gave his subjects bread and butter, milk and a helping of meat and potatoes and then recorded the intra-sigmoid pressures for the next 35 to 40 minutes. Such an ordinary meal was often followed by the generation of complex pressure waves whose base-line was raised for two to three minutes and upon which a succession of peaks of pressure greater than 30 mm. of water were superimposed. Sometimes waves exceeding 50 mm. of water followed each other in quick succession. These waves were only seen in

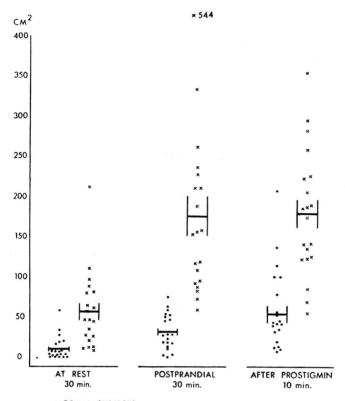

FiG. 43. The distribution of pressures in health and diverticulosis. Eating and prostigmine increase the pressures in the colon but this effect is much greater in patients with diverticulosis than in healthy subjects. The transverse lines represent the mean values and the standard deviations are indicated. Other investigators have reported that prostigmine evokes a much greater response than does eating; it is possible that different methods of investigation and of calculating the total pressure produced may account for these different findings. (Reproduced from Arfwidsson, 1964, by kind permission.)

diverticulosis and were never observed in the normal colon. In ten subjects with diverticulosis, the total intrasigmoid pressure was increased postprandially by more than six times than that seen in normal subjects and waves exceeding 30 mm. of water were nearly six times as frequent in the diseased colon as in the normal.

These pressures were significantly different from those seen prior to taking a meal and the pressures in the diseased bowel were statistically different from those in the normal. Arfwidsson concluded that, in diverticular disease, the sigmoid was prone to produce high pressures and that, as a consequence, the daily act of feeding would tend to favour the progression of the disease once it had become established. This effect of the 'gastro-colic reflex' has been observed since by Attisha and Smith (1969) and by Smith and his colleagues (1971). The postprandial pressures are not as great as those which follow prostigmine but their effect presumably is felt by the colon throughout life (Fig. 44). Parks (1970), using air-filled balloons, found that postprandial pressures in diverticulosis were only slightly greater than in the healthy colon and Parks and Connell (1972) observed less mean pressure in the diseased than in the

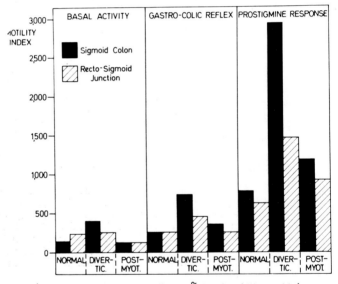

(Motility Index = Mean Wave Amplitude X % Duration of Wave Activity)

Fig. 44. Response of sigmoid colon and recto-sigmoid in health and in diverticular disease to feeding and prostigmine. (The diagram shows the mean motility indices depicted for basal activity, the effect of the gastrocolic reflex and of prostigmine; motility index = mean wave amplitude $x\%$ duration of wave activity).

The 'gastrocolic reflex' calls forth an increase in the pressures generated by the sigmoid which is not as great as that evoked by prostigmine. This effect is more marked in patients with diverticular disease. The 'post-myotomy' columns reveal that Reilly's operation of sigmoid myotomy reduces the intracolonic pressure; this operation is described later in this book. (From Smith *et al.*, 1964.)

healthy colon after food, even though more waves of high pressure were generated by the diseased colon during the times that it was active. The observations of various investigators differ because some used balloons instead of open-ended tubes and some gave prostigmine intramuscularly and others administered the drug intravenously. Tracings described from balloons relate to the pressure in the balloon which varies with the extent to which it is buffeted by the bowel wall and do not measure the intraluminal pressure.

This differential response of the diseased colon to the intake of food is of the greatest importance as it shows that a natural stimulus which occurs frequently can lead to the generation of high intrasigmoid pressures in diverticular disease.

(6) THE EFFECT OF EMOTION

It has been known since the earliest times that emotion and, in particular, fear or anxiety may affect the bowel and cause abdominal pain or even involuntary defaecation. The motility of the colon has been shown to alter in response to pain and to anxiety felt by volunteers in the course of experiments (Almy, Kern and Tulin, 1949; Almy, Hinkle, Berle and Kern, 1949; Almy, Abbott and Hinkle, 1950). The effect of anxiety was seen frequently by the author in the Nuffield Institute for Medical Research when he was filming the movements of the colon during continuous pressure recording. The sound of the x-ray machine being switched on immediately prior to filming often affected the patient sufficiently to stop all pressure production so that the tracing became flat almost immediately even though it had been active up to that moment. Occasionally, this sound would be followed by the appearance of pressure waves on a previously 'flat' tracing. These patterns of colonic activity appeared to be due to hidden anxiety in patients who were outwardly calm.

Colonic motility may alter in response to the broaching of an unpleasant topic. A lady of 45 volunteered to have her colon pressures investigated. Once the tubes were in position and she was resting on a bed, she was engaged in conversation in order to put her at her ease. She mentioned that her daughter was a nurse who had become engaged to a patient who was suffering from tuberculosis. She disapproved strongly of this match and feared for her daughter's future. While she talked, she was completely unaware of the increased activity of her colon (Fig. 45). This topic was referred to again later when her colon was

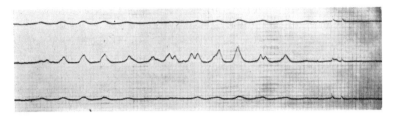

FIG. 45. The effect of emotion on the pressures in the sigmoid colon. Pressures recorded from the sigmoid colon of a lady of 45. Pressure waves of up to 40 mm./ Hg were recorded when the subject discussed an unpleasant topic; for description see Chapter 8. (From Painter, 1962.)

still and generating no pressure waves. Her colon became more segmented almost immediately and produced a series of pressure waves of up to 40 mm./Hg in amplitude during the ensuing conversation (Painter, 1962). This phenomenon was seen on several occasions and was so striking that one laboratory technician suggested the use of intracolonic pressure recording as a form of 'lie detector'. What role emotion plays, if any, in the production of the disease is unknown. On clinical grounds, it seems possible that it may play a subsidiary role in that it alters colonic motility and this may be important in patients whose bowel motility is already disturbed or is being subjected to some other stress such as an abnormal diet.

(7) THE EFFECT OF MECHANICAL FACTORS

The colon may be stimulated by the injection of only 1 c.c. water into its lumen. Such a quantity was often injected into the bowel through the open-ended polythene tubes either when they were being filled at the beginning of the recording session or when they had become blocked with faecal matter and were being cleared with a few c.c.s of water. The injection of this small quantity of fluid was usually followed by waves of pressure of up to 10 mm./Hg in amplitude for a few minutes following the injection.

This effect was even more apparent when the bowel had been

activated by morphine or prostigmine. Painter (1962) delib-
erately injected 10 c.c. of a fine barium suspension (micropaque)
into the sigmoid in health and diverticulosis while filming the
behaviour of the bowel. The diseased bowel might generate
pressures of 20 mm./Hg in response to this stimulus and, after
morphine, the injection of a few c.c.s into the lumen near
diverticula sometimes evoked pressures of over 90 mm./Hg.

These observations show that the movement of fluids within
the healthy and more especially in the diseased sigmoid may
result in the generation of high pressures. It has been observed
clinically that the administration of purgatives and enemas in
diverticulitis is sometimes followed by perforation and it seems
possible that this is due to pressures evoked by a similar stimulus.

(8) THE EFFECT OF OTHER DRUGS

Painter (1962) gave 50 mg. of dihydrocodeine bitartrate (DF.
118) intramuscularly to three healthy patients. The colonic
pressures were raised very slightly. Phenazine (Narphen) in a
dose of 2 mg. intramuscularly was given to two healthy patients
with no apparent effect on the basal patterns of pressure.
Probanthine given after DF. 118 stopped all pressure generation.
The investigation of such small numbers proves nothing but
suggests that further experiments might show that these drugs
would be safe to give to patients with colonic diseases.

(9) THE PRESSURES IN THE 'PREDIVERTICULAR STATE'

Spriggs and Marxer (1925) coined this term to describe the
narrow sigmoid which appeared to be shortened by contraction
of the longitudinal muscle so that it was thrown on to folds like
a concertina. These changes precede the appearance of diverticulosis. Such sigmoids are difficult to fill with barium and tend to
reject barium so that they are said to be spastic. Edwards (1934)
and Morson (1963) showed that the colonic muscle may be
thickened and show all the changes of diverticulosis except that
no diverticula are present. These observations are most important and suggest that these muscular changes may be accompanied by alterations in the normal pattern of pressures before
the actual herniation of the mucosa takes place.

Arfwidsson (1964) therefore recorded the pressures in colons, showing these radiological changes at rest, after food and after prostigmine. He found that both eating and prostigmine increased the total intracolonic pressure nearly five times while pressure waves of greater than 30 mm. of water in amplitude occurred five times as frequently after food and nearly six times as often after prostigmine in comparison with those in the normal colon. Painter and Truelove (1964) demonstrated a differential response to morphine in a patient with only one demonstrable diverticulum; this patient's colon is shown in Fig. 53. Parks (1970) recorded pressures in descending colons which had been anastomosed to the upper rectum after resection of the sigmoid for diverticulitis and found that prostigmine elicited greater pressures from this part of the bowel even though it was free of diverticula.

These observations support those of Arfwidsson and confirm that abnormal pressure patterns are present before diverticula appear. Diverticula appear to be only the outward visible sign of some earlier abnormality of colonic motility.

(10) THE SIGNIFICANCE OF THESE PRESSURE STUDIES

Accurate recording of the intraluminal pressure reveals that the basal pressure in the resting colon is the same in health as it is in diverticulosis. Hence, the disease is not caused by 'intraluminal hypertension'.

Segments beset with diverticula respond differently when activated by morphine and prostigmine by producing higher pressures and produce more total pressure than do normal segments. From a practical standpoint, the wisdom of giving morphine in acute diverticulitis must be questioned as it evokes high pressure that may predispose to perforation; its effect on colonic anastomoses may also be harmful (Painter and Truelove, 1963).

Pethidine (demerol) has not this disadvantage and it appears to be the analgesic of choice in colonic disease.

Prostigmine given at the end of an operation may jeopardize the integrity of colonic and ileo-rectal anastomoses (Bell and Lewis, 1968; Wilkins, Hardcastle, Mann and Kaufman, 1970).

This differential response of the diseased segments is of great theoretical interest, as it suggests that once the disease is established, it is liable to progress. The diseased sigmoid reacts excessively to naturally occurring stimuli such as emotion and eating, the latter occurring regularly every day, and so it seems inevitable that the diseased segments generate and have to withstand higher pressures than does the neighbouring bowel.

The demonstration by Arfwidsson (1964) that the contracted colon in the 'pre-diverticular state' produces excess pressures leaves little doubt that high intrasigmoid pressures precede the appearance of diverticula and that the latter are not the primary abnormality, a view supported by the observations of Painter and Truelove (1964b) and of Painter, Almeida and Colebourne (1972).

The significance of the colon's ability to localize high pressure near to the tip of one recording tube, so that another only 7·5 cm. distant fails to register any alteration of pressure, will be discussed in the next chapter as will the mechanism by which probanthine abolishes the generation of intra-colonic pressure waves.

Chapter 9

The Segmentation Mechanism of Pressure Production

Two questions arise from the various pressure studies that have been described in Chapter 8. First, how does the colon produce pressures which can be localized to the vicinity of the tip of one recording tube while another tip only 7·5 cm. distant is unaffected by these pressures? Second, what effect do the high pressures that are evoked by morphine and other stimuli have on diverticula? The first question will be dealt with in this chapter and the second will be discussed in Chapter 10.

Open-ended tubes record the pressure at their tips continuously and accurately. They give no information as to the movements of the bowel and they cannot differentiate between pressures which are generated by activity in close proximity to their tips from those pressures that owe their origin to events occurring at a distance. Hence, open-ended tubes record pressures accurately but throw little light on the mechanism responsible for their production. The use of simultaneous cineradiography makes it possible to link the configuration of the colonic wall and the state of the diverticula with any changes in the intraluminal pressure that may occur. This chapter describes the results obtained by this method.

METHOD OF COMBINING CINERADIOGRAPHY WITH PRESSURE RECORDING

Painter and Truelove used intermittent cineradiography combined with continuous pressure recording; the equipment they used was described by Ardran and Wyatt (1954 and 1957). Briefly, an image intensifier coupled to an electron lens enabled a 5 in. diameter image to be photographed on to 35 mm. film. Each volunteer was subjected to less than six roentgens which is about one tenth of that involved in a diagnostic barium enema examination. Exposures were made at 1 frame per second and, as each frame was taken, the tracing was marked by a pen. This enabled the appearances of the bowel, which was outlined by barium, to be correlated with the pressure tracing. The position of the metal-capped tips of the recording tubes were visualized radiologically while the contour of the sigmoid colon was delineated by its contained barium. The colon was photographed at rest, when active and while it was being influenced by drugs. During these experiments, the patient rested on a stretcher. On occasions, the patient was filmed with his right side nearest to the camera if a still film of the abdomen showed that loops of the sigmoid overlapped each other (Painter, 1962; Painter, Truelove, Ardran and Tuckey, 1965b).

When the films had been developed, they were spliced in a loop and then projected at varying speeds so that the activity of the colon could be studied repeatedly at leisure. The appearance of the bowel in each frame was studied in conjunction with the pressure tracing in order to elucidate the means by which the colon produces high localized pressure.

(2) THE SEGMENTATION MECHANISM OF PRESSURE PRODUCTION

(a) As a means of Producing Localized Pressure

The similarity of the form of the successive waves that follow the administration of morphine suggests that they are produced by the same mechanism. Recording pressures at three levels in the bowel simultaneously shows that the colon can localize pressure so that a high pressure recorded by one lead does not affect another situated only 7·5 cm. away (Fig. 31). In the absence of any obstruction by foreign bodies and faeces, it is obvious that the colonic wall must be responsible for this localization of pressure and cineradiography showed this supposition to be correct. When high waves of pressure were generated, it was found that the colon was not functioning as the open tube depicted in text books of anatomy, but as a series of segments separated by contraction rings. This 'segmentation mechanism' was shown to build up pressures and localize them to a segment of the colon.

Consider the colon as an open tube characterized by haustral markings in the top diagram of Fig. 46. The slight movements of its wall that have been shown to occur by balloon studies and

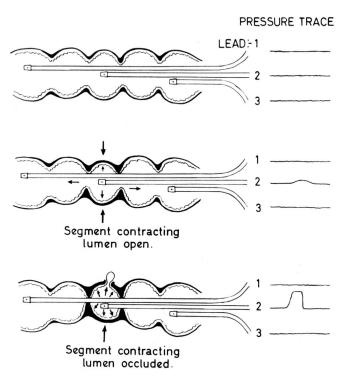

FIG. 46. Diagram to show segmentation causing high pressures and the pulsion force responsible for diverticulosis. Diagram shows three longitudinal sections of colon with three open-ended pressure recording tubes (or leads) in position. The top section shows that, as long as the lumen is open, small movements of the bowel wall will not cause any significant pressure change, as the contents of the bowel are free to move. In the middle section, the centre segment is demarcated by two contraction rings that narrow the lumen on each side of it. Further contraction of the centre segment will be resisted by its contents, as they cannot flow freely into the neighbouring bowel, and a pressure change will be recorded by lead 2 that will not affect the segments on either side. The bottom longitudinal section shows that the centre segment contracted so that the lumen on each side of it is almost occluded. Further contraction of the segment would cause a very high pressure to develop and would be recorded by lead 2, but the leads on either side of it would not record a pressure change, as the bowel around them is open. It is obvious that the centre section is behaving as a 'little bladder' in which high pressure can develop, and it is this pressure that causes the extrusion of the mucous membrane between the contraction rings. (From Painter, 1964.)

by cineradiography will disturb its fluid contents and cause them to move without let or hindrance, other than the resistance offered by their viscosity, to another part of the colon. Thus, the muscle coat has little resistance offered to its contraction and only a slight and transient alteration of the intracolonic pressure will occur. These recording leads in such a colon will record no significant change of pressure; this is depicted on the right of the diagram.

A different state of affairs is shown in the middle diagram of the same Figure. The middle segment is partly shut off from its neighbours by contraction rings. This segmentation narrows the lumen of the bowel on each side of the segment so that, when it contracts, its contents are no longer entirely free to move into the neighbouring segments. A rise of an intraluminal pressure will occur if the wall of this segment contracts and moves its contents against the resistance offered by the contraction rings. This pressure will fall only when the segment ceases to contract or its contents escape. The middle lead will record a wave of pressure as shown on the right of the diagram. Leads 1 and 3 will be unaffected by these events as they are situated in open bowel where the colonic contents are free to move.

The fully developed stage of the process is seen in the bottom diagram. The middle segment is completely isolated from its fellows by contraction rings which have occluded the lumen on each side of it. If this segment now contracts, it will compress its contents if they are gaseous but if they are solid or liquid, and therefore almost incompressible, it will contract isometrically. In either event the resultant rise in pressure will be steep as the contents cannot escape from the segment. A recording lead in this segment will record a wave of high pressure which will be limited to this segment and will not affect the 'open' segments in its neighbourhood. This bottom diagram of Fig. 46 represents the extreme limit of the segmentation mechanism. This is shown in the frames of cine-film reproduced in Figs. 47 and 48; one is of a normal colon and the other shows a diseased colon segmenting.

(b) Segmentation Promoting the Transport of Colonic Contents

Figure 49 illustrates how segmentation is involved in initiating the movement of colonic contents. A segment, isolated from its fellows by contraction rings, may raise the pressure within

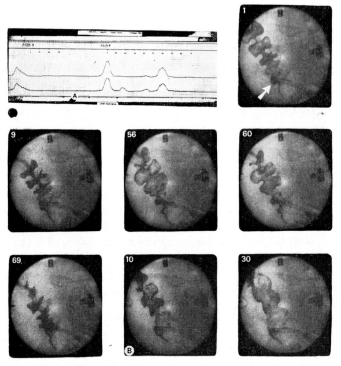

Fig. 47. *A*, Film of a normal colon which had segmented in response to Prostigmin; two pressure waves were recorded while filming. *Frame 1* shows the tip of the recording lead (arrowed in frame) was in segmented bowel as a pressure of 78 mm. Hg was recorded in the upper tracing. This pressure had fallen to the base line by *frame 9* and the bowel around the tip had relaxed so that the segment containing it was in free communication with the lumen of the bowel below. The pressure was again rising when *frame 56* showed that the colon was again segmenting about the tip, which was in a contracted segment when a pressure of 50 mm. Hg occurred (*frame 60*). Thereafter the bowel relaxed so that this segment came into free communication with the bowel below (*frame 69*). Concurrently the pressure fell. This film showed that when pressures followed the use of Prostigmin, their generation was accompanied by segmentation. *B* shows two frames taken later when the pressure remained at the base line for several minutes; in both, the colon was widely open about the tip (from Painter *et al.*, 1965.)

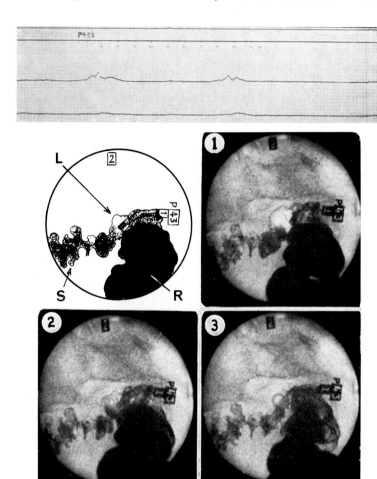

FIG. 48. The production of pressure by segmentation. The diagram shows the rectum (R) and sigmoid (S) of a patient with diverticulosis. The tip of a recording lead (L) is situated in a segment of the sigmoid. This segment was relaxed when it only harboured the basal pressure (Frame 1), but when it contracted, in an attempt to propel barium up the bowel, the pressure within it rose to 6 mm. Hg (Frame 2). As it contracted further, this pressure rose to 20 mm. Hg (Frame 3). The upper pressure tracing is derived from lead (L) and the left-hand wave of pressure resulted from the contraction of the segment that contained this lead, and the frames shown relate to this wave of pressure.

it by the mechanism described above until it exceeds that harboured by neighbouring segments. If one contraction ring then relaxes, the contents of the segment will flow into the adjoining bowel where the pressure is less. This action may be likened to that of a Higginson syringe. The further movement of these contents will then depend on the behaviour of the segments into which they have passed.

THE SEGMENTATION MECHANISM CAUSING
———————— TRANSPORT ————————

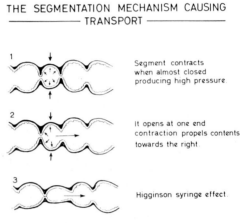

1 Segment contracts when almost closed producing high pressure.

2 It opens at one end contraction propels contents towards the right.

3 Higginson syringe effect.

FIG. 49. Diagram to show how pressure localized to one segment may be utilized to initiate the movement of the colon's contents.

(c) Segmentation Limiting the Movement of Colonic Contents

The ability of the colon to occlude its lumen enables it to stop the flow of matter within it, be it gas fluid or solid. This may be achieved by one contraction ring or by a succession of rings acting as a series of baffles, each of which retards the onward movement of colonic contents until, finally, they are halted (Fig. 50).

(d) Functions of the Segmentation Mechanism

So far the role of only a single segment has been discussed so as to keep the description simple, but several segments may act together so that material is moved back and forth in the colon. The segmentation mechanism is capable of initiating or stopping the transport of colonic contents in either direction.

The symmetry of the colonic segments allows them to propel, receive, pass on or halt the colon's contents in either direction.

THE SEGMENTATION MECHANISM STOPPING
———————— TRANSPORT ————————

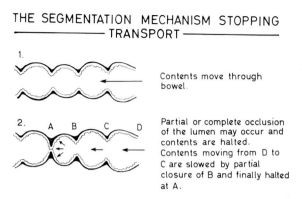

1.

Contents move through bowel.

2. A B   C   D

Partial or complete occlusion of the lumen may occur and contents are halted. Contents moving from D to C are slowed by partial closure of B and finally halted at A.

FIG. 50. Diagram to show how segmentation can halt material which is moving through the colon.

This enables the sigmoid to shunt material back and forth, presumably in connection with the absorption of water from the faecal stream. Painter (1967) and Painter and Burkitt (1971) have pointed out that stiff faeces resulting from an abnormal diet require greater pressures to initiate their transportation and suggested that half a lifetime of being subjected to pressures that are abnormal either in amplitude or in their frequency of occurrence causes the colon to develop diverticulosis. The sigmoid would be subject to the greatest strain as its contents are more viscous than are those of the proximal colon and this may be why the sigmoid is the site of election of diverticular disease.

(3) SEGMENTATION—THE COMMON FACTOR IN THE PRODUCTION OF LOCALIZED PRESSURES

The recognition of the role of segmentation in the genesis of intracolonic pressures was facilitated by studying the colon after it had been activated by morphine and prostigmine. Cineradiography revealed that both these drugs cause the colon to segment so that its lumen is narrowed at intervals. Further contractions of the colon converts it from an open tube to a series of 'little bladders', each of which may generate and harbour a pressure which is localized to this segment, and which differs from the pressure in neighbouring segments. Both drugs cause the colon to segment so that, when it becomes active at intervals, high pressures are generated. In between bouts of activity following the use of these drugs, the sigmoid stays segmented but no pressures are generated until the segmental wall between the inter-haustral folds contracts.

Cineradiography revealed that when pressure waves were recorded the colon always became segmented in the vicinity of the tip of the recording tube. This was true, whether pressures arose spontaneously as a result of food or emotion or following the administration of morphine or prostigmine. No doubt other mechanisms may exist that produce pressures but Painter *et al.* (1965a) failed to observe any mechanism that did not involve segmentation.

Rarely, the bowel may close down so that its lumen is occluded for several inches. This corresponds to the state of the colon that is loosely described as 'spasm' by radiologists. It may equally be regarded as an extreme degree of segmentation in which several neighbouring segments have contracted concurrently to such an extent as to convert the colon into a straight tube whose lumen has been obliterated temporarily.

By contrast, pethidine which reduces the number of waves of high pressures and the total pressure also lessens the degree of segmentation. At the same time the drug renders the colon less active and less susceptible to a physical stimulus such as injecting barium into its lumen (Figs. 51 and 52). Probanthine which abolishes the production of intracolonic pressure, including even the high pressures evoked by morphine and prostigmine, achieves this result by paralysing the colonic muscle. Cineradiography shows that probanthine causes the colon to relax so that it becomes an inert tube with a wide lumen and, as it relaxes, so does the production of pressure cease (Fig. 55), (Painter, 1962 and 1964; Painter *et al.* 1965a and b).

These observations show conclusively that the intracolonic pressures are generated by local activity of the colonic musculature which produces pressure by contracting after partially occluding the colonic lumen. Therefore, any stimuli which encourage segmentation will increase the total intracolonic pressures, and any drugs which cause the colon to relax so that its lumen is widened will lessen these pressures. It would appear that it is possible to predict the effect of a new drug on the pressures in the sigmoid by administering the drug during the course of a barium enema examination. If the drug accentuates

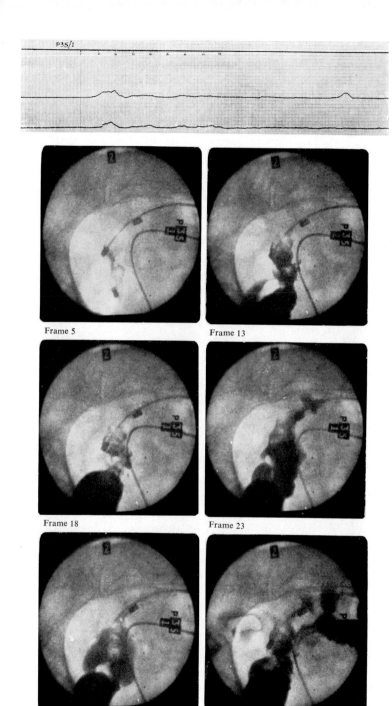

FIG. 51. The effect of an injection of barium into the colon in diverticulosis (for details see Chapter 10).

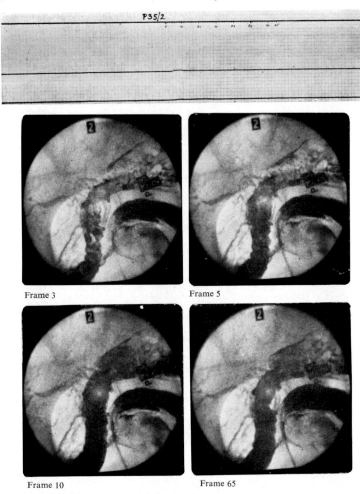

Frame 3   Frame 5

Frame 10   Frame 65

FIG. 52. The effect of an injection of barium into the lumen of the colon in diverticulosis after the administration of pethidine (for details see Chapter 10).

the degree of segmentation it may be expected to raise the intraluminal pressures whereas a drug that relaxed the bowel would probably have the reverse effect.

Once it was realized that the living colon does not function as the tube that is depicted in anatomy text books but as a series of 'little bladders', the reason for the similarity of colonic and vesical diverticula became clear. Bladder diverticula result from chronic partial obstruction of the bladder neck, while colonic diverticula are caused by intermittent functional obstruction of the outflow of the colonic segments. The thickening of the muscle coat of the colon that is characteristic of diverticular disease may be compared with the trabeculation seen in the urinary bladder.

Chapter 10

The Effect of Drugs in Diverticular Disease of the Colon and the Role of Segmentation in the Pathogenesis of Diverticula

The pressure studies described in Chapter 8 show that the diseased colon generates very high pressures near diverticula when activated by certain stimuli, including morphine and prostigmine. Whether these pressures were transmitted to the actual diverticula was at first uncertain but cineradiography revealed that these pressures distended the mucosal pouches, a process that would predispose to their rupture. The evidence presented in this chapter leaves little doubt that morphine is potentially dangerous if used as an analgesic in acute diverticulitis and that pethidine does not have its undesirable effects.

Segmentation is responsible for the production of intracolonic pressures (Chapter 9), and its role in the pathogenesis of diverticula will be described in this chapter.

(1) THE EFFECT OF MORPHINE, PROSTIGMINE, PETHIDINE, PROBANTHINE AND MECHANICAL STIMULI ON DIVERTICULAR DISEASE OF THE COLON

(a) Morphine

Morphine sulphate given intramuscularly has been shown to increase the total pressure produced by the colon in health and in diverticulosis. Painter and Truelove (1964a) found that waves of high pressure were evoked by morphine in segments of the colon which bear diverticula. Such segments sometimes generate a succession of pressure waves in excess of 90 mm./Hg and they suggested that the use of morphine as an analgesic in acute diverticulitis might favour perforation of the inflamed mucosal sacs. They realized that contraction of the necks of diverticula might protect them from these high pressures and so they used cineradiography to study the effect of the drug in sigmoid colons that were beset with diverticula.

Fig. 53 shows the sigmoid colon of a woman of only 58 in which only one diverticulum was demonstrated. The tip of a recording tube situated in the lumen adjacent to the neck of the diverticulum recorded two waves of 20 mm./Hg and 30 mm./Hg. The cinefilm showed that the neck of the diverticulum remained open and the diverticulum became better filled. As the pressure rose, barium was seen to be squeezed into the diverticulum which was outlined as a bifid shadow suggesting that it contained a faecolith. This shows that diverticula are subject, at least in part, to the pressures produced by morphine (Painter *et al.*, 1965b).

Sometimes, morphine produces dramatic changes in diverticula. Fig. 54 shows the sigmoid of a woman of 70 years old which was so serpentine that its loops overlapped each other in the film and, for this reason, it was impossible to pass more than one recording tube above the recto-sigmoid junction. Hence, the intraluminal pressure near the two diverticula which are seen in the right lower quadrant of the printed frames was not recorded. However, pressures of up to 20 mm./Hg were recorded from the bowel below the diverticula after the intravenous injection of morphine was made, being completed by the 21st frame of the film.

The necks connecting these two diverticula to the lumen of the colon are clearly seen in frame 20. The intravenous morphine sulphate took effect, almost immediately and the bowel began to narrow rapidly in the next ten seconds. Simultaneously, the diverticula enlarged (frame 30) and their necks narrowed until, at times, they were shut completely (frame 50). The bowel from which they arose contracted so that its lumen was almost occluded (frame 60). When this film was projected, the activity of the colon increased greatly after morphine and the diverticula appeared to be blown up like balloons. Although the necks of the diverticula closed at times (frame 95), they opened intermittently (frame 99) and allowed barium to be pumped into the mucosal sacs.

This was not a temporary effect, as was shown by a film taken 40 minutes later of the same subject (Fig. 55). Consequently, there is little doubt that morphine is contra-indicated for the relief of pain in acute diverticulitis. The drug increases the activity of the colon and its excitability with regards to the movement of even 1 c.c. of fluid in its lumen and so morphine

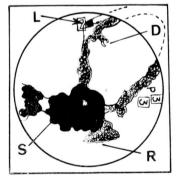

Frame 10

Frame 25

Frame 38

Frame 42

FIG. 53. The effect of morphine on the colon in diverticulosis (for details see text). D = diverticulosis, L = lead 2, R = rectum, S = sigmoid (for description, see text of this chapter).

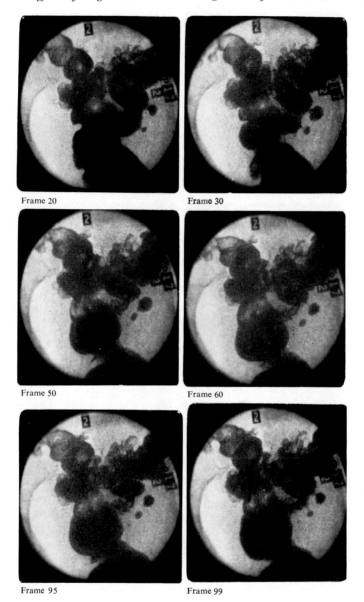

Frame 20 · Frame 30 · Frame 50 · Frame 60 · Frame 95 · Frame 99

FIG. 54. The effect of morphine on colonic diverticula (for details see text of this chapter).

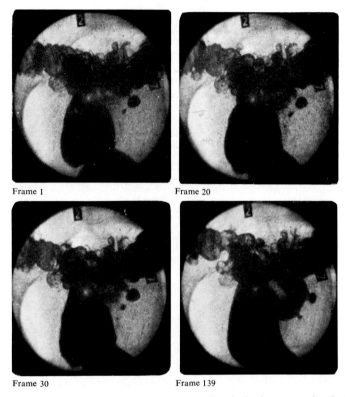

Frame 1   Frame 20

Frame 30   Frame 139

FIG. 55. The effect of probanthine on colonic diverticula that are under the influence of morphine (for details see text of this chapter).

does not rest the injured colon. The distension of diverticula by morphine is dramatic. Pethidine (demerol) has the opposite effect; it relaxes the colon and opens the necks of diverticula so that their contents can drain into the bowel. Pethidine lowers the intracolonic pressure and is the analgesic of choice in acute diverticulitis. The author will not prescribe morphine in acute diverticulitis or after colonic anastomosis and Reilly (personal communication), regards the drug as dangerous both before and after myotomy.

(b) Prostigmine

Prostigmine has an effect similar to that of morphine and cineradiology shows that it achieves its effects by increasing segmentation. Like morphine, prostigmine elicits a differential response from the affected segments and distends diverticula (Fig. 56). This observation is not of mere theoretical interest as its use by anaesthetists may account for the disruption of ileo-rectal and other anastomoses (Bell and Lewis, 1968; Wilkins *et al.*, 1970).

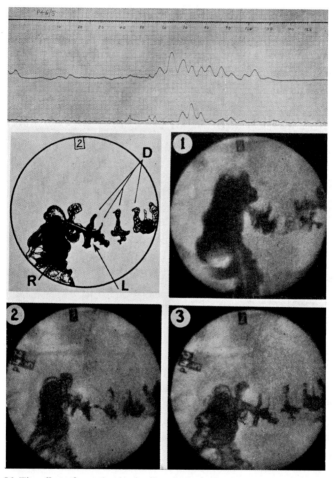

FIG. 56. The effect of neostigmine in diverticulosis. Pressure tracing shows a wave of 60 mm. Hg occurring after neostigmine. This was recorded by a lead (L in diagram) in the sigmoid whose tip was in the immediate vicinity of diverticula (D). Before this wave of pressure, the diverticula were small (frame 2), but they were distended by this wave of pressure (frame 3). Frame 1 shows the bowel before neostigmine had been given; in this cinefilm, the sigmoid was less seg-mented and the diverticula were seen to fill better as their parent segments con-tracted. (From Painter, 1964.)

(c) Pethidine (Demerol)

Pethidine lessens the degree of segmentation, the total pressure generated and the frequency of occurrence of waves of high pressure; both in health and in diverticulosis. It appears that it achieves this effect by diminishing the excitability of the colon so that it does not segment in response to stimuli that normally excite it. Fig. 51 shows the reaction of the sigmoid of a woman of 64 years with diverticulosis to an injection of barium into its lumen. Frame 5 shows the metal tips of three polythene tubes in the colon; that farthest up (lead 1) recorded pressure as did the lowest tube tip (lead 2). In between them a 'feeder' tube (lead F) was situated and this was used to inject barium into the colon without interrupting the recording of pressures by leads 1 and 2. 20 ml. of barium was injected between the second and twelfth frames of this film. As it passed up the sigmoid, the bowel segmented around lead 1 and produced a wave of 19 mm./Hg (frames 13 and 18). Two diverticula enlarged as the pressure rose and are seen on the right hand side of the bowel. A second injection of barium was made between the 26th and 33rd frames; most of it flowed to the rectum, being unable to pass up the sigmoid which had by now segmented (frames 23, 30 and 40). The bowel again reacted to this second injection by segmenting.

Figure 52 shows the same bowel after pethidine. The tips of the recording tubes can be recognized through the shadows cast by the barium that had been injected as has been described (frame 3). Barium was injected via lead F between the third and tenth frames and it was seen to pass along the sigmoid in either direction like water flowing through an open drain (frames 5, 10 and 65). The passage of this barium was not hindered by any sudden alteration in the configuration of the bowel wall, neither did its lumen narrow and nor did contraction rings form. In short, the colon did not segment or produce pressure in response to the same stimulus that previously had caused it to react vigorously. After pethidine, the diverticula appeared as squat projections with open necks which was quite unlike their appearance in the previous figure. Obviously, pethidine affects the sigmoid so that it does not react to stimuli that normally excite it, and this supports the view that pethidine should be given as an analgesic in colonic disease as it 'rests' the bowel and does not endanger the integrity of infected diverticula.

(d) Probanthine

Probanthine in a dosage of 15 mg. or 30 mg. abolishes the pressures produced by the colon whether they occur spontaneously or after morphine or prostigmine. The drug paralyses the colon within 15 to 20 seconds of being given intravenously and within 12 to 15 minutes of being injected intramuscularly, both in health and in diverticulosis (Fig. 42). It converts the colon into an inert tube with a wide lumen on which the haustral markings are less distinct. This effect lasts for up to three hours during which no pressures are produced. Figure 55 shows the same colon of the woman of 70 that has been described (Fig. 54). After 40 minutes, morphine still caused the colon to be contracted and 30 mg. of probanthine was given intravenously; this was completed by the 11th frame. The diverticula in the right lower quadrant were distended (frame 1) but, during the next 130 frames taken at one frame per second, the sigmoid and the diverticula changed dramatically. The motor activity of the bowel ceased and it dilated and pressure generation ceased. As the sigmoid became wide and immobile, the necks of the diverticula opened and allowed the contained barium to drain into the bowel so that they diminished in size. To sum up, probanthine reverses the sequence of events that follow the use of morphine.

The ability of probanthine to relax the colon has been used by Lumsden and Truelove (1959) as an aid to the diagnosis of colonic lesions. The drug blocks the transmission of impulses by the autonomic nervous system when used in this dosage; this effect suggests that morphine may act through autonomic pathways which supports the suggestion of Vaughan Williams and Streeter (1950) that a central mechanism is involved when morphine acts *in vivo*. While this is of theoretical interest, probanthine given intramuscularly might be of practical value in the treatment of acute diverticulitis; a trial of the drug in this condition is long overdue. Side effects such as dryness of the mouth and loss of visual accommodation would be of little inconvenience to patients confined to bed, but the danger of prolonging ileus must be borne in mind. Meanwhile, pethidine should be used as it has some of the effects of probanthine. Oral probanthine given as a relaxant for the relief of colonic pain is prescribed frequently but there is no evidence that it is of benefit.

(2) THE ROLE OF SEGMENTATION IN THE PATHOGENESIS OF DIVERTICULA

(a) Segmentation causing the Pulsion Force responsible for Diverticulosis

Colonic diverticula are similar in structure to the diverticula which are commonly found in the urinary bladder which has had to struggle for many years to void its contents through a partially obstructed bladder neck. The striking resemblance between the two types of diverticula was at once apparent to the earliest investigators of diverticular disease and, as a consequence, they were puzzled to find no obvious anatomical hindrance to the passage of the faecal stream (Gross, 1845; Bristowe, 1854). Naturally, they looked for some form of organic obstruction to account for the presence of diverticula but their post-mortem studies only revealed a thickened colon beset with diverticula whose lumen, while it might be narrowed, was not obstructed.

In retrospect, it is only too obvious that these writers, who so accurately predicted the cause of diverticulosis, were handicapped by the limits imposed by the technology of their time. They could only examine inert dead tissues and so the pathogenesis of diverticula remained a mystery until the advent of cineradiography. This made it possible to examine the living human colon and revealed that, when segmented, it assumes a configuration that leads functionally, if only intermittently, to its own partial or even complete obstruction. Cineradiography showed that segmentation divides the colon into a series of 'little bladders', each of which has its outflow obstructed at each end. The contraction of any one of these isolated segments or 'bladders' results in the generation of high localized pressures that distend diverticula arising from these segments (Figs. 56 and 57). The actual extrusion of diverticulum from a sigmoid colon whose lumen narrowed and segmented in response to an injection of morphine was filmed by Painter (1962). There is little doubt that segmentation is responsible for the pulsion force which displaces the colonic mucosa (Painter, 1962 and 1964; Painter *et al.*, 1965b).

(b) The Nature of the Contraction Rings Seen in Segmentation

The recognition of the relationship between segmentation and the pathogenesis of diverticula revealed that the colonic muscle

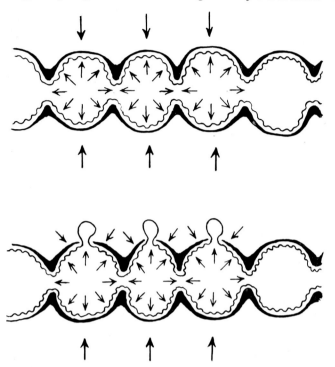

FIG. 57. Diagram to show how segmentation produces the pulsion force that distends colonic diverticula, and probably causes the initial mucosal herniation.

can contract differentially so as to form contraction rings between the colonic segments. Whether these contraction rings always occur at the same place is still uncertain. The author carefully scrutinized cine-films of the diseased colon, taken both before and after the administration of drugs, and observed that diverticula arose without exception from the wall of the segments between the contraction rings and never originated from the contracted inter-segmental folds. Using the diverticula, which were fixed in position, as reference points, the contraction rings appeared to form always at the same site. This observation is in keeping with the claim of Poirier and Charpey (1914) that the muscle between the haustra is greater in amount and is consistent with Edwards's histological studies which also provide an anatomical basis for the differential contraction of the colonic muscle that is seen in segmentation.

However, at the present time, there is no direct evidence to show that these rings always form at the same site in the normal colon. Pace and Williams (1969) dissected the colonic muscle coat and failed to find any evidence of there being any structural basis for segmentation. Recently, Hodgson (1972) produced reducible diverticula in rabbits by feeding them a low residue diet and noted that these diverticula always appeared at the same site.

These observations are not so incompatible as they appear at first sight. It may be that these fibres of the circular muscle, which are responsible for forming the contraction rings, cannot be differentiated from their fellow fibres on histological grounds as far as the normal colon is concerned, and that it only becomes possible to differentiate them microscopically in the abnormal colon. It seems obvious that these fibres alter in response to the abnormal stimulus that causes diverticulosis and that they have already altered in the 'pre-diverticular state' described by Edwards. Certainly, the site of these contraction rings is fixed in the advanced stages of the disease when the muscle has bunched into reduplicated folds between which the colonic wall contains little or no muscle fibres and hence cannot contract. The author believes that the contraction rings which demarcate the colon into segments always occur at the same sites and that the structural basis for this only becomes visible after some abnormal stimulus has caused the muscle fibres of the contraction rings to hypertrophy. This results in the uneven thickness of the muscle coat in which bands of circular muscle become apparent histologically. In the final fully developed stage of the disease the sites of contraction are marked by thick folds of muscle and are obviously constant in position.

Much more work is needed before the process is fully understood, but it seems to be similar to the hypertrophy of muscle fibres which is seen in the urinary bladder. It is likely that the changes which are so characteristic of diverticular disease are the result of 'trabeculation' of the colonic 'bladders' brought about by excessive segmentation.

(c) Segmentation and the Diameter of the Colon

Segmentation produces high localized pressures by narrowing the colonic lumen so that it is partially or completely obstructed. When a colon, whose diameter is wide, segments, its lumen does not become functionally obstructed to the same extent as does that of a colon which is narrow *ab initio*. The small bore colon is more efficient in producing high pressures as its lumen can be obstructed more readily. This may be one reason why the sigmoid, which is the narrowest part of the colon, is the site of election of diverticulosis (Painter, 1964).

The diameter or bore of the colon varies with the diet. The West African native eats a diet which contains plenty of fibre and which produces a large residue. He has a colon of wide diameter and does not suffer from diverticular disease (Wells, 1949; Painter and Burkitt, 1971). Similarly, the colons of rats fed on a bulk-forming diet remain free of diverticula and have a wide lumen. Conversely, the colons of rats and rabbits fed on low residue diets become narrow and develop diverticula (Carlson and Hoelzel, 1949; Hodgson, 1972). It would appear that the size of the colonic lumen, and hence its ability to generate high pressures, can be altered by a long-acting stimulus. It is therefore possible that not only the nature of the diet but other long-term stimuli, such as the taking of laxatives, may also affect the size of the colon. In the short term, the stimuli that evoke localized intracolonic pressures also cause the colon to narrow. This applies to natural or mechanical stimuli and to drugs such as morphine or prostigmine.

Segmentation is more efficient in narrow colons. Hence, anything which narrows the colon, either in the long or the short term, will be of aetiological significance as far as diverticulosis is concerned.

(3) CONCLUSION

Segmentation is responsible for the localized pressures that cause diverticulosis. Hence, drugs and other stimuli which cause segmentation also increase the intracolonic pressure. On the other hand pethidine, which lessens the degree of segmentation, reduces the pressure generated by the colon and probanthine, when given in a dosage which paralyses the colonic muscle, abolishes the production of all pressure waves in the colon.

Cineradiography combined with intraluminal pressure recording shows that diverticula are caused by pressures produced by the active contraction of the colonic muscle and not by passive distension of the large bowel.

The administration of morphine and prostigmine is followed by very high intraluminal pressures which can distend diverticula to an alarming degree. Consequently, the use of morphine for the relief of pain in acute diverticulitis is contraindicated as it may lead to perforation of the mucosal sacs. Pethidine appears to be the analgesic of choice in acute diverticulitis because it lowers the intraluminal pressures and lessens the excitability of the colon so that it does not have this undesirable effect.

It seems likely that prostigmine, if used by anaesthetists at the end of operations, may threaten the integrity of anastomoses that involve the large bowel.

The pathogenesis of diverticular disease involves segmentation. Hence, any hypothesis which seeks to explain the appearance of diverticula must take account of segmentation or it will be untenable.

Chapter 11

The Epidemiology and Aetiology of Diverticulosis and its Relationship to Dietary Fibre

INTRODUCTION

Diverticular disease of the colon was unknown at the turn of the century, but it has since become the commonest affliction of the colon in the Western world. Historical, epidemiological and clinical studies support the view that the condition is caused by the removal of vegetable, and in particular cereal, fibre from the diet. At the time of writing, diverticular disease of the colon has the unique distinction of being the only common disease whose symptoms have been relieved by the replacement of the fibre that is missing from our modern diet.

Although the present incidence of diverticulosis is unknown, it is certainly extremely prevalent in our aged citizens. The disease has appeared as a clinical problem and its incidence has increased dramatically in only 70 years. Theoretically, this change can only be explained in three ways. First, it might be due to a genetic change in the whole population but this idea is too ridiculous to contemplate seriously. Second, this change may be due to observer error and hence be more apparent than real but the quality of their writings, some of which have been reported in Chapter 2, shows that the clinicians of the last century were just as capable as those of today of recognizing diverticulitis had it been common in their day. A third possibility remains, namely, that the colon's environment has been changed and that diverticula are caused by our modern diet and, in particular, by changes in that fraction of it which reaches the colon.

THE HISTORICAL EMERGENCE OF DIVERTICULITIS AS A CLINICAL PROBLEM

The history of this common disease has been considered in Chapter 2. Diverticula of the colon were recognized and, together with their complications, were described in detail in the last century. However, they remained a curiosity of no clinical significance until the early nineteen-hundreds when diverticulitis appeared on the clinical scene as a surgical emergency. Like appendicitis, it took surgeons by surprise at first but by 1920 it had become recognized as a 'newly discovered bane of elders' (Telling and Gruner, 1917; Bland–Sutton, 1920).

When radiological methods of examining the bowel came into general use after the First World War, it was found that diverticula were much commoner than had been thought and attempts were made to discover the true incidence of this 'new' condition. Necropsy studies showed that diverticula were rare before the age of 40, confirming that they are an acquired abnormality. Necropsy and barium enema estimates of the prevalence of diverticulosis are given in Tables 12 and 13. Both methods of investigation have their faults; autopsies are performed on more old subjects and barium enemas are usually undertaken for symptoms. Radiological series exaggerate the incidence of diverticulosis while necropsy findings vary with the personal interest of the pathologist in disorders of the colon. The true incidence of the disease could only be found by subjecting a sample of the population to annual barium enemas but, obviously, this is not practicable.

When due allowance has been made for these limitations, it seems that Mayo (1930) was probably very near to the truth when he estimated that 5% of colons in patients over the age of 40 bore diverticula, as this figure agrees with contemporary necropsy series in the United States and Britain. Barium enemas were used more sparingly in those days but yielded a similar incidence of 4–10% and this appears to have increased but little in the next ten years. Morton (1946) reviewing American autopsies and Edwards (1953) quoting English barium enema studies, recorded similar figures.

The incidence of diverticulosis has obviously risen dramatically in the United Kingdom, the U.S.A., Australia and France in the last 20 years. Between one half of those over the age of 40 have diverticula and this incidence rises to two thirds at 80 years (Parks, 1968; Hughes, 1969). The disease must have become commoner in Australia in the last 20 years as it was much less frequently found there in the 1940s (Cleland, 1968).

Diverticular disease of the colon was almost unknown in 1900,

TABLE 12

INCIDENCE OF COLONIC DIVERTICULA: NECROPSY SERIES

Country and Author	Incidence of Diverticula		No. in Series	Comments
	%	No.		
United Kingdom:				
Drummond (1917)	4·4	22	500	London Hospital, 55% of subjects were under age 30, so incidence over 40 would probably have been 5%
Fifield (1927)	2·1	—	10,167	
Parks (1968)	37	111	300	Northern Ireland, 50% in ninth decade
United States:				
Hartwell and Cecil (1910)	5	—	81	New York, 1909–10
Rankin and Brown (1930)	5·6	111	1,925	All but one subject aged over 40
Oschner and Bargen (1935)	6·9	—	447	All necropsies in one year
	3·58	—		Over age 40
	15·2	—		White women over age 70
Kocour (1937)	7·1	—	7,000	White men over age 70
	2·0	—		Coloured man over age 70
	3·0	—		Coloured woman over age 70
Morton (1946)	6·3	—	8,500	Rochester, N.Y.
Australia:				
Cleland (1968)	2·6	78	3,000	Refers to 1940–8. Incidence rose with age
	6·2	36	589	Over age 70 in this period
Hughes (1969)	45	90	200	43% if caecal diverticula excluded

but has become the commonest affliction of the colon in Western countries within only 70 years, the traditional life span of man.

THE GEOGRAPHICAL DISTRIBUTION OF DIVERTICULAR DISEASE

(a) General Remarks

This dramatic rise in the prevalence of diverticulosis has occurred only in the industrialized countries of the Western world whose diet has changed only recently in the time scale of human nutrition. There are few diseases whose incidence varies so much throughout the world as that of diverticulosis, namely, from nil to nearly 30% of a population. This incidence is closely related to the degree of economic development and to the degree to which the diet has altered as a consequence of the introduction of food processing. The prevalence of the disease also varies with the degree of the social changes that have occurred in those countries which presently are altering their way of life and corresponds to that which pertained in the Western countries at a similar stage in their industrial development when the pattern of their life was similar. Obviously, due allowance has to be made for the fact that this acquired disease takes about 40 years to develop, even after the colon's environment has been changed. Therefore, diverticulosis would not appear in a community until it had departed from its traditional eating habits for half a lifetime. Consequently, the disease will not be prevalent in a country until the unfavourable effects of economic progress with its concurrent dietary changes have been felt for 40 years. Thus the disease would be expected to be almost unknown in sub-Saharal Africa to this very day and this is indeed the case.

The greatest contrast in the incidence of diverticulosis is to be seen between the Western world, including North American Negroes, and rural Africa and Asia. Countries which have only recently altered their pattern of life have an intermediate incidence; the disease is three times as common in highly industrialized Sweden as it is in Finland (Kohler, 1963).

This relationship between the prevalence of the disease and the degree to which the local diet has changed in recent years, was established by enquiries made by post and by personal visits over the past five years (Painter and Burkitt, 1971).

TABLE 13

INCIDENCE OF COLONIC DIVERTICULA: BARIUM ENEMA SERIES

Country and Author	Incidence of Diverticular		No. in Series	Comments
	%	No.		
United Kingdom:				
Spriggs (1920)	0·6	6	1,000	Mainly adult patients. Importance of post-
Spriggs and Marxer (1925)	10	100	1,000	evacuation film had been realized
Edwards (1934)	10·8	—	507	Period 1925–31, King's College Hospital. Patients aged over 40
Grout (1949)	8	—	2,179	Relates to previous 13½ years and all patients
Edwards (1953)	16	25	1,623	over age 35
Manoussos et al. (1967)	7·6	—	109	7·6% below age 60 Deliberate study by Ba
	34·9	—		34·9% over age 60 meal and follow-through in normal people
Sweden:				
Lunding (1935)	4·2	87	2,090	
France:				
Debray et al. (1961)	40	—	500	40% over age 70. All patients had gastro-intestinal symptoms
United States:				
Enfield (1924)	1·2	—	—	Found incidentally on barium studies
Mayo (1930)	5·71	1,819	31,838	Mayo Clinic

Rankin and Brown (1930)	5·67	1,398	24,620	Mayo Clinic
Oschner and Bargen (1935)	7	—	2,747	Enemas given for intestinal symptoms
Willard and Bockus (1936)	8·2	38	463	Consecutive enemas in private practice
Eggers (1941)	7·5	—	647	Barium meal followed through colon
	44·5	—	428	Barium enemas
Allen (1953)	30	—	2,000	Enemas given for symptoms. No diverticula under age 35, 5% at 45, 66% in older age groups
Welch et al. (1953)	8·5	—	47,000	Collected series; 66% incidence over age 80
Smith and Christensen (1959)	22	—	1,016	Consecutive enemas. Years 1954–8; incidence doubled at 80 years

(b) Diverticular Disease in Africa

The native population of Africa were little affected by the Industrial revolution which occurred in the Western countries just over a century ago and enquiries reveal that diverticular disease is almost unknown in rural Africa to this very day. Mr Denis Burkitt practised surgery in Africa for 20 years, mostly in a teaching hospital, and did not encounter a single case of diverticulitis, nor did his colleagues see the disease. In South Africa, Keeley (1958) found no diverticula in 2,367 autopsies between 1954 and 1956 performed at the 2,000 bed Baragwarath Hospital, Johannesburg, which serves the most urbanized Africans. At the same hospital, Solomon (1971) found six cases in about 1,000 barium enemas performed in Bantu patients over a three year period. Levy (1972) saw no diverticula in over 100 enemas given to urbanized Africans in 13 years and Bremner and Ackerman (1970) stated that the Bantu practically never get diverticulosis. At Pretoria, Simpson (1972) found the disease only five times in 3,000 autopsies performed with great care on Bantu, Chapman (1971) saw one case in an African in 14 years at the King Edward VII teaching hospital in Durban.

According to Trowell (1960), Davies at Kampala, Uganda, performed 4,000 autopsies in 15 years and found two diverticula, while Templeton (1970) carefully scrutinized 300 colons from Africans over the age of 30 and found only one case of the disease in an African woman of 80 whose sigmoid was affected. Miller (1971) saw diverticulosis in an African only once during 11 years at the Kenyatta Hospital, Nairobi. Professor Hutt (1970) saw none in his department of pathology in eight years. Jain (1971) working at a medical school at Kinshasha, in Zaire, saw one case in nine years. At the medical school in Accra, Ghana, Bado (1971) saw one patient with the condition in 16 years. Calder (1971) saw one patient with diverticulosis in two and a half years in Malawi.

Kyle *et al.* (1967) recorded that only two cases of diverticulitis were seen in the University Hospital at Lagos in three years. The first example of diverticular disease in a Rhodesian African was reported by Wapnick and Levin (1971). Goulston (1967) stated that diverticulosis was infrequent and diverticulitis was unknown in Ethiopia.

Admittedly, it could be argued that diverticulosis might be

missed where facilities are limited but it is inconceivable that diverticulitis, which presents as a surgical emergency and often leads to death, could remain unrecognized in major African hospitals with first-class staff, equipment and extensive necropsy experience. There is no doubt that the disease is extremely rare even in the large teaching hospitals that cater for the most urbanized Africans, so it is not surprising that enquiries addressed to doctors in over 150 mission and up-country hospitals in Africa confirm that diverticular disease is, for practical purposes, unknown in rural Africans.

(c) The Indian Sub-Continent and the Middle East

Even in urban communities in these regions the disease is still rare.

Delhi. Bhardwaj (personal communication, 1973) found only five cases in 9,000 barium enema examinations and Bhargaua (personal communication, 1973) has seen only 12 cases in 15 years in a department performing 600 barium enemas a year and all were found in 'Westernized' Indians.

Calcutta. Banerjee (personal communication, 1973) diagnoses the disease less than once a year out of more than 300 barium enemas.

Iraq. Mahommed Abu-Tabikh (personal communication, 1973) reports that about 1,000 barium enemas are performed annually in the University Hospital, Baghdad, and diverticula are detected in no more than three cases.

Iran. Zaraki (personal communication, 1971) saw five cases of diverticular disease in the teaching hospital at Shiraz where 500 enemas are performed annually. All five patients belonged to the top socio-economic group.

(d) Diverticular Disease in the Far East

The disease is almost as rare in Asia as it is in rural Africa. Tinckler saw ten cases in one and a half million Chinese, Indian and Malayan inhabitants of Singapore in five years, but three in 15,000 Europeans (Kyle *et al.*, 1967). In Kuala Lumpur, Malaysia, Kutty (1970) found no diverticula at autopsy in three years and de Beaux saw only a single case among 137,000 native Fijians as against two in the 7,500 resident Europeans; the Europeans were relatively young and passed as physically fit before going to Fiji (Kyle *et al.*, 1967). Kim (1964) found no diverticula in 500 autopsies in Korea. Plenyvanit (1972) detected diverticula twice in 91 barium enemas performed in Bangkok. Anderson (1970) and Wright (1970) did not see the disease in India and New Guinea respectively.

In Japan, diverticulosis was rare but has appeared, mainly in males, in Tokyo in the last six years according to Doctor Chikai Yazana who reported this to the International Conference of University Colon and Rectal Surgeons at Rhodes, 1972; 1,987 barium enemas had shown diverticula in 131 patients (6·6%) in the ratio of three males to one female.

It is often suggested that some of these countries have fewer elderly citizens than do the industrial countries but this could not affect the issue sufficiently to account for the almost complete absence of the disease in the developing countries. This is especially so as in recent years diverticula are appearing by the age of 35 in Europe and America in increasing numbers.

This survey confirms that diverticular disease is rarely found in peoples whose eating habits have changed but little up to the present, while it is extremely common in the industrial nations where food is processed and refined.

(e) Changes in Incidence following Dietary Changes within a country or on Emigration

Some 40 years ago, diverticular disease was much less prevalent in American negroes than it was in their white compatriots (Kocour, 1937) but this difference has almost disappeared. During the same period the black American has become more affluent and his diet has become similar to that of white Americans, while the sale of maize for human consumption has fallen (Cleave, Campbell and Painter, 1969).

Until recently the disease was almost unknown in Japan, but the disease is very common in Japanese who have been born and bred in Hawaii and who were reared on a Western diet (Stemmerman, 1970 and personal communication, 1972). The few cases which have been recorded in India and Iran have, for the most part, been in the top socio-economic groups who tend to eat Western-type foods.

Similarly, diverticulosis affects West Indians who have lived in Britain for many years although, like the American Negro, they are of the same stock as the rural African who is free from the disease. Obviously, diverticulosis is not due to any difference in race.

DIETARY FIBRE AND DIVERTICULAR DISEASE

In theory, the amount of fibre in the diet may be reduced not only by the refining of flour and cereals but also by the substitution of refined sugar for unrefined foodstuffs that were previously eaten. In practice, these two processes occur together as both follow industrialization which necessitates the growth of towns and the need for food supplies to be transported from a distance. This, in turn, is followed by the need to preserve foodstuffs in warehouses which is facilitated by refrigeration and by the refining of cereals.

In Britain, the diet changed dramatically around the years 1870–1880. Stoneground white flour had been freely available since 1800, (McCance and Widdowson, 1956) but a daily diet of 21 oz. (600 g.) of stoneground wheat mixed with rye, together with oatmeal porridge was not uncommon in the poorer classes as late as 1860. Much of the fibre had been removed by stonegrinding but in 1870 the introduction of roller milling removed almost all the fibre that remained in our flour. This was accompanied by a fall in the consumption of bread as alternative foods became cheap so that our intake of fibre derived from grain has fallen so that today it is only one tenth of that consumed in 1870.

During the same years, improvements in rail and sea transport and the use of refrigeration made other foods available. The ending of the American civil war allowed the grain and meat of North America to be brought to Europe and chilled meat began to arrive from Australia, New Zealand and South America. The value of British wages rose by 30% in ten years and the import tax on sugar was reduced (Barker, McKenzie and Yudkin, 1966). As a result meat imports doubled and the consumption of refined sugar and jam, which is 60% sugar, almost doubled between 1865 and 1890 (Cleave, Campbell and Painter, 1969). Since then, canning and refrigeration have made more and more perishable foodstuffs available to the public out of season.

These changes resulted in an increase in the intake of fat and protein and a corresponding fall in the consumption of bread and products made from flour. This fall in the consumption of bread has continued to the present day except for the years of the two world wars when bread was made from flour of higher extraction. Consequently, the greatest change that has occurred in the British diet is the dramatic fall in the amount of dietary fibre ingested, the very part of our food which reaches the colon with the least change.

If this swing from a high- to a low-fibre diet is responsible for diverticulosis then the disease, which takes half a lifetime to develop, would be expected to be prevalent about forty years after 1880 and, in fact, diverticulosis was common in Britain by 1920.

These changes are similar to those which took place in the U.S.A. in this century when the increasing prosperity of the American Negro led to a fall in the consumption of maize and a rise in the incidence of diverticulosis among black Americans (Cleave, Campbell and Painter, 1969; Painter and Burkitt, 1971). The same dietary differences can be found in the Japanese who live in Japan and those who migrated to Hawaii and the continental United States.

I believe that around 1880, the British diet was depleted of fibre sufficiently to damage the colon. The evidence suggests that the refining of flour and cereals is the primary cause of diverticulosis, while the consumption of refined sugar at the expense of bread further increased the loss of dietary fibre. Admittedly, much bran had been removed from flour before this date, but it would appear that the colon has so far failed to adapt to this further fall in dietary fibre that has occurred in the last century.

At this very moment, the diet of Africans living south of the Sahara is changing rapidly but they have not eaten a low-residue diet for long enough to cause them to suffer from diverticulosis. It has been postulated that appendicitis is caused by eating refined carbohydrates (Short, 1920; Cleave, Campbell and Painter, 1969; Burkitt, 1971; Walker *et al.*, 1973) and so if both appendicitis and diverticulosis are caused by fibre-deficiency, then appendicitis which is becoming increasingly common in urban Africans will be followed by the appearance of diverticulosis after a time interval similar to that which separated their recognition in Britain. Close observation of these dietary changes and the altering incidence of disease in this part of the world may well reveal the causation of these and other diseases.

THE RELATIONSHIP OF DIETARY FIBRE TO THE PATHOGENESIS OF DIVERTICULAR DISEASE

If a deficiency of dietary fibre causes diverticulosis, this must be related to colonic segmentation which is the mechanism responsible for the mucosal herniation. The role of segmentation in colonic physiology and in the genesis of diverticula has been discussed in Chapters 9 and 10.

It is suggested that an unrefined diet containing adequate fibre may prevent diverticulosis for the following reasons:

(1) The colon that copes with a large volume of faeces is of a wider diameter and does not develop diverticula. This is true in man (Wells, 1949) and experimental animals such as rats (Carlson and Hoelzel, 1949) and rabbits (Hodgson, 1972a). Such a colon having a wide bore *ab initio* segments less efficiently than does a narrow colon and is less prone to diverticulosis (Painter, 1964).

(2) Studies of transit times and stool weights are described in Chapter 22. In most instances, the food residue passes through the African gut within 48 hours whereas, in an Englishman, this may take twice as long (Hinton *et al.*, 1969; Burkitt *et al.*, 1972). Thus, the African's colon absorbs water for less time and so has to propel a less viscous faecal stream. Hence, the African's colon has to do less work and produce less pressure by segmentation; his colon is thus less likely to become "trabeculated" and to bear diverticula than is a colon that has to struggle for many years with the viscous contents that result from a low-residue diet.

(3) In Western countries custom often demands the suppression of the call to stool which favours the drying of faeces and increased pressure generation. On the other hand, the South African Bantu can pass large motions on demand without straining (Walker *et al.*, 1970).

In short, the swiftly passed soft stool subjects the sigmoid to less strain and does not favour the development of diverticula.

ORIGIN OF THE LOW RESIDUE DIET IN THE TREATMENT OF DIVERTICULAR DISEASE

The low-residue diet, which was the mainstay of the medical management of diverticulosis for nearly 50 years, was founded on a misunderstanding of the cause of the condition. Spriggs and Marxer (1927) believed that constipation and the stagnation of faeces in the sigmoid led to infection which weakened the colonic wall. Consequently, they gave paraffin to cleanse the colon and enough fruit and vegetables to make the stools soft and bulky. Undigested fragments of vegetable stalks and bone had been found near to perforated diverticula (Cripps, 1888; Bland-Sutton, 1903; Brewer, 1907) and, unfortunately, this was interpreted as evidence that these foreign bodies had caused the perforation and subsequent peritonitis. Consequently, a low-residue diet, free of fibrous stalks and pips, and in which all fruit and vegetables were made into a purée, was advocated by authorities such as Slesinger (1930); Oscher and Bargen (1935); Willard and Bockus (1936); Brown and Marcley (1937); and by Harold Edwards (1939). Dimock (1936) recorded that Lord Dawson of Penn pronounced that 'roughage' irritated the gut. What was not digested was 'indigestible' and was considered, quite erroneously, to be the cause of indigestion.

In retrospect, it is quite remarkable that the low-residue diet was adopted by the profession as a whole despite the lack of any evidence to show that it was of any benefit and that in nearly 50 years no trial was reported which demonstrated the efficacy of this regimen. The wisdom of prescribing a low residue diet was questioned by Painter (1962) and by Painter *et al.* (1965a). Painter and Burkitt (1971) stated that this diet is contra-indicated in the treatment of diverticular disease because it is the cause of the condition.

THE TREATMENT OF UNCOMPLICATED DIVERTICULAR DISEASE BY A HIGH FIBRE DIET

If a deficiency of dietary fibre causes diverticulosis, it is logical to replace the fibre in the diet. Painter, Almeida and Colebourne (1972) gave unprocessed bran to 70 patients with uncomplicated diverticulosis who were complaining of symptoms. They found that a high-fibre/low-sugar diet relieved or abolished 88·6% of the symptoms complained of by 70 patients. This regimen of treatment and their results are discussed in Chapter 21. Whether a high-fibre diet will prevent future attacks of painful diverticular disease or acute diverticulitis is not yet known but there is little doubt that it is very effective in relieving or abolishing even severe colic which could otherwise only be treated by major surgery.

ANIMAL FEEDING EXPERIMENTS THAT BEAR ON DIVERTICULAR DISEASE

Carlson and Hoelzel (1949) fed rats on a high residue diet and they did not develop diverticula, while those who were fed on a low-residue diet had a contracted colon which bore diverticula. They proposed that their narrow colon, which resulted from a low-residue diet, was more prone to become obstructed at the acute angle where the rat's colon joins the rectum and that this partial obstruction caused diverticula to develop. Painter *et al.* (1965a) suggested that this could be explained in another way, namely, that the narrow colon could segment more efficiently and so produce higher pressures and diverticula. Recently, Hodgson (1972a) fed six New Zealand white rabbits on white bread, butter, milk and sugar supplemented by vitamins. He measured the intracolonic pressures before and after prostigmine prior to giving this diet and afterwards. This 'refined diet' caused the rabbits to gain weight while their general condition deteriorated and they became constipated. Their colons narrowed and the administration of prostigmine caused scattered wide-necked reducible diverticula to appear. The total pressure produced by the colon when activated by prostigmine was increased after the colon had been altered by this diet. His findings were essentially similar to those reported in humans by Painter (1962, 1964) and by Painter *et al.* (1965b). These experiments lend support to the view that a low-residue diet is the cause of diverticulosis even though they must be interpreted with caution if only because of the different life span of the species investigated.

THE EFFECT OF A HIGH RESIDUE DIET ON THE INTRACOLONIC PRESSURES IN MAN

Hodgson (1972b) gave methyl-cellulose (celivac) to six patients with diverticular disease for six months and recorded the pressure in their colons before and after feeding. He concluded that the intracolonic pressures were reduced by the addition of methyl-cellulose to the diet; all six patients became symptom-free on this regimen. This small series offers some support to the view that a soft faecal stream stimulates less pressure production, but it would be a pity if methyl-cellulose, which has been known to clump and cause obstruction, were to be used in diverticular disease when bran, which is not only natural but has been shown to be safe, is readily available at a price that even the poor can afford.

Recently, Adam Smith (1973) reported the effects of bran on the intracolonic pressures after sigmoid myotomy. Reilly's operation has been shown to reduce the intracolonic pressures and to widen the lumen of the colon while relieving symptoms (Smith, Attisha and Balfour, 1969; Smith, Giannakos and Clarke, 1971) but these pressures rise again in about two years if the patient keeps to his previous diet. Therefore, Smith instructed patients who had undergone myotomy to take the 'bran diet' and found that, after three years, the reduction in intracolonic pressures had been maintained (Smith, 1973). His observations can be explained on the grounds that, if the diet is not changed after operation, then the factor that produces diverticulosis is still operating. No urologist would allow an aniline dye worker who had developed a papilloma of his bladder to continue in his employment; he would treat the local disease and alter his environment. The same applies to diverticular disease. Surgery, whether it takes the form of resection or of myotomy, is only an incident that deals with the complications of the disease; hence, it is logical to suggest that these operations should be followed by the taking of a high-fibre diet so that the underlying cause of the condition is removed.

CONCLUSION

Historical, epidemiological and clinical studies provide abundant evidence that diverticulosis coli is a disease that has become common in economically developed nations who eat a diet in which the carbohydrates are refined. Feeding rats or rabbits with a low-residue diet lends support to this view. The replacement of dietary fibre has been shown to diminish or abolish the symptoms of the established disease and to prolong the beneficial effects of sigmoid myotomy.

All these observations suggest that much more attention should be paid to the amount of fibre, and in particular cereal fibre, in our diet. Diverticular disease and its complications are an increasing problem in Western countries and there is every reason to believe that the appearance of the disease could be prevented. It is worth remembering that the rise in the death rate from diverticular disease was halted in Britain only during the war and immediate post-war years when white bread was not available and refined sugar was strictly rationed (Fig. 58). Perhaps a return to this diet would achieve more than all our surgical endeavours. It is the duty of the profession to point the way to prevention, even if it means warning against the dangers of such popular foodstuffs as white flour, both brown and white sugar, confectionary, and food and drinks which contain unnaturally concentrated carbohydrates.

Diverticular disease is a deficiency disease and, like scurvy, it should be avoidable. By retracing our dietary footsteps so that fibre is retained in our food, it should be possible to prevent the appearance of the disease in future generations and, also, to lessen the incidence of cancer of the colon which has a similar epidemiology.

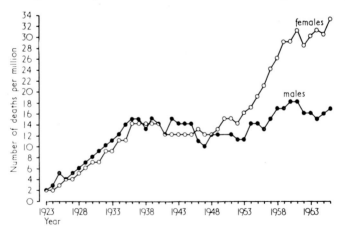

Fig. 58. Crude death rate for diverticular disease: Registrar General's statistical review of England and Wales 1923–66. (From Cleave, Campbell, and Painter, 1969.)

Chapter 12

The Clinical Manifestations of Diverticular Disease of the Colon: their Classification, Traditional Treatment, and Prognosis

INTRODUCTION

The clinical manifestations of diverticular disease of the colon are many. They vary from vague dyspepsia to unheralded acute abdominal pain and to peritonitis which, even to this day, is often lethal. The majority of patients with the condition lead normal lives, while others only suffer from 'indigestion', flatulence, a feeling of distension, lower abdominal discomfort or an abnormal bowel habit. Together, these patients constitute the bulk of those with diagnosed and undiagnosed diverticulosis and they usually remain under the care of their family doctor. Most of them are unaware of the existence of their diverticula and so mild forms of the disease are seldom discussed in text books.

It is indeed fortunate that the disease is so seldom incapacitating because the minority of those who have diverticula suffer from recurrent attacks of abdominal pain or colic and an unlucky few of them are smitten by true inflammatory diverticulitis and its dreaded complications. This small portion of those with the disease present as very difficult problems which often need prolonged hospital treatment. Consequently, it is the surgical management of the complications of diverticulitis that has attracted most attention in the literature.

As diverticular disease may be discovered incidentally, or may make its presence felt in such a variety of ways, it is essential that its manifestations are classified before their presentation can be discussed and a rational approach to their treatment can be considered.

In an attempt to satisfy these conditions, the nomenclature used in this book is one of recent origin. It differs from the traditional classification which divided the disease into 'diverticulosis' and 'diverticulitis'. This change became inevitable when Morson (1963) showed that, even in the absence of inflammation, the diseased sigmoid could cause pain of a severity sufficient to lead to partial colectomy and when Painter (1962; 1964 and 1968) suggested that the colic of so-called 'diverticulitis' could be caused by excessive segmentation of the colon.

THE TRADITIONAL DIVISION OF THE DISEASE INTO 'DIVERTICULOSIS' AND 'DIVERTICULITIS'

When the disease was first recognized, it was thought that the diverticula were the primary abnormality and that they were responsible for any symptoms that appeared to originate in the colon. Originally, by definition, diverticulosis meant that diverticula were present but were not inflamed and were not causing symptoms. Conversely, it was axiomatic that patients who complained of abdominal discomfort or pain and who had diverticula, but no other demonstrable disease, were suffering from 'diverticulitis'. This traditional division of the disease into diverticulosis and diverticulitis was founded on the incorrect premise that diverticula were the primary abnormality and it had several unfortunate results.

First, it compelled doctors to place their patients into one of two categories. Hence, a diagnosis of 'diverticulitis' was made if patients with diverticulosis complained of symptoms whether or not they had fever and even when their white cell count was normal. This makes the interpretation of much of the earlier literature of diverticular disease very difficult and renders some of the older communications almost valueless. Often, the reader cannot be sure whether patients were operated on for colonic pain or for inflammatory diverticulitis and so he cannot always compare the experience of the last generation of writers with that of today's clinicians.

Second, radiologists were expected to find radiographic evidence of diverticulitis in any patients who were referred to them while complaining of symptoms. This they did with such remarkable ingenuity that many papers were published in which radiologists claimed that uncomplicated diverticulosis and diverticulitis could be differentiated by means of a barium enema. It is now known that many of the radiographic signs that were said to distinguish diverticulosis from diverticulitis are not due to inflammation and that the differentiation of uncomplicated diverticulitis from diverticulosis by barium enema is unreliable. It has been realized recently that such radiographic features as the 'pre-diverticular state', 'pallisade', 'saw toothed' or 'serrated' colons are caused by the muscle changes that precede and accompany the presence of diverticula and that they should not be interpreted as reliable evidence of inflammation (Fleischner, 1971).

The limitations of radiology in differentiating between diverticulosis and diverticulitis were made abundantly clear by Parks and his colleagues (1970). They compared the initial x-ray diagnosis with the clinical presentation and subsequent course of 461 patients with symptomatic diverticular disease, of whom 90% required admission to the Royal Victoria Hospital, Belfast, between 1951 and 1965. By chance, 230 were said to have 'diverticulosis' and 231 were diagnosed by barium enema as suffering from 'diverticulitis'. However, when the previous history presenting symptoms and signs, pattern of bowel habit, incidence of complications and later treatment were analysed, no significant difference was demonstrated between the two groups. Even the application of modern diagnostic criteria failed to improve the correlation between x-ray reports and the final pathological diagnosis. The Belfast group showed beyond doubt that radiology is almost useless in detecting the presence of uncomplicated diverticulitis and is of no help in assessing the immediate or future clinical state of patients.

Thirdly, it led to the introduction of the 'low residue diet'. As even the mildest symptoms used to be attributed to 'diverticulitis' whose complications were so feared, it seemed eminently reasonable to both physicians and surgeons to forbid any food that might cause diverticula to become inflamed. This led to the introduction of the 'low residue diet' in the mistaken belief that roughage irritated the colon and might perforate diverticula. This diet remained in vogue for nearly 50 years until it was realized that it failed to relieve and often exacerbated the symptoms that it was intended to prevent.

THE TRADITIONAL TREATMENT OF UNCOMPLICATED DIVERTICULOSIS

When contrast radiology revealed that colonic diverticula were common even in people who had no symptoms, the term 'diverticulosis' was coined to distinguish this state of affairs from the recently recognized disease of diverticulitis. As the complications of diverticulitis were dangerous and diverticula were so dramatic when demonstrated by barium enema, it was almost inevitable that the profession felt that it was its bounden duty to treat them, notwithstanding the fact that their aetiology was unknown. Hence, it is scarcely surprising that a regimen for the conservative treatment of diverticulosis appeared in the text books where it remained virtually unaltered for nearly half a century.

Spriggs and Marxer (1925) believed that diverticula protruded from a sigmoid that had been weakened by infection due to the stagnation of its contained faeces and so they gave gentle enemas and mineral oil to cleanse the colon. Very soon afterwards, physicians, in the mistaken belief that roughage irritated the gut and that fragments of bone and the stalks of vegetables had been responsible for perforating diverticula, began to advocate a 'low residue diet' in which all fruit and vegetables were reduced to the consistency of today's canned baby foods.

The former attitude of the profession was discussed by Horner (1958) who remarked that some doctors regarded diverticulosis as a harmless anatomical disorder that at the worst was amenable to medical treatment while others thought it to be the precursor of diverticulitis and that it must be treated. He thought that most gastroenterologists agreed that uncomplicated diverticulosis was asymptomatic but that custom decreed and 'experience has shown it to be sound practice, for patients to avoid foods that leave rough undigested particles in the stool'. The stools were kept soft with small nightly doses of mineral oil, mucilage or wetting agents. 'Patients who are willing to accept the discipline of this dietary programme rarely develop difficulty. Those who do suffer an attack of diverticulitis are usually quite aware of the offending article of diet' (Horner, 1958). The grounds on which they confidently identified this article of their diet were not specified.

The traditional treatment of diverticulosis consisted of giving liquid paraffin and a low residue diet from which all pips, seeds, stalks and the fibrous parts of fruits and vegetables were rigidly excluded. Constipation was to be avoided but strong purgatives were forbidden. Some recommended gentle enemas but others discouraged their routine use (Barborka, 1958; Botsford and Curtis, 1961).

Mild symptoms were attributed to a 'spastic' or 'irritable' colon or to diverticulitis. Horner (1958) had strict criteria and considered that diverticulitis should only be diagnosed if fever was present and the white count was raised, but others assumed that any symptoms were caused by diverticulitis but that the degree of inflammation might be so mild that no constitutional upset, alteration in the white cell count or change in the sedimentation rate could be detected (Feldman and Morrison, 1949). Episodes of pain were treated medically with rest, paraffin, low pressure enemas, belladonna, hyocyamus and the application of local heat. A low residue was prescribed once the attack of pain had subsided. In later years, the sulpha drugs and antibiotics, together with probanthine, were also used therapeutically (Slesinger, 1930; Willard and Bockus, 1936; Edwards, 1939; Laufman, 1941; Horner, 1958).

For nearly 50 years this regimen was accepted despite the fact that no controlled trial of its efficacy was ever published and no convincing evidence was ever produced that it was of any benefit. Both Case (1928) and Mayo (1930) believed that the colon had to struggle with a low residue diet and it is now known that such a diet is contraindicated in the treatment of the disease because it is caused by fibre deficiency (Painter and Burkitt, 1971). In retrospect, it seems certain that the traditional treatment of diverticulosis was harmful. The author has been assured by several patients who had adhered consistently to a low residue diet that not only did it fail to relieve their symptoms but it made them worse. All were relieved when they changed to a high fibre diet including unprocessed millers' bran. A few of them who returned to a low residue diet as a temporary experiment reported that their symptoms returned.

These adverse effects of the low residue diet did not escape the notice of some clinicians. Certainly, several had abandoned its use more than ten years ago and were advising their patients to eat whatever they wished even though the standard text books still advocated a low residue diet. Long before the disease was attributed to fibre deficiency, others were prescribing Kellogg's All-Bran to keep the bowels open daily and the stools soft (Harold Dodd—personal communication, 1969).

The low residue diet was given a fair trial for nearly 50 years but experience showed that it was of no benefit.

THE ORIGIN OF SYMPTOMS IN UNCOMPLICATED DIVERTICULAR DISEASE

Although at first all symptoms were interpreted as being evidence of diverticulitis, it was soon realized that patients with colonic diverticula and an otherwise normal alimentary tract often complained of abdominal pain and discomfort when no clinical signs of any inflammatory process were detectable. Moreover, symptoms were difficult to attribute to diverticula if only because they included flatulence, fullness, vague dyspepsia and generalized abdominal discomfort which appeared to be of upper intestinal origin.

Whether uninflamed diverticula could cause symptoms became a subject for debate (Hughes, 1970). Feldman and Morrison (1949) considered this problem and, realizing that these symptoms did not always bear a temporal relationship to episodes of proven diverticulitis, attributed the symptoms of no less than 63% of 205 patients with diverticulosis to an 'irritable' or 'spastic' colon. Likewise, Fagin (1955) tried to ascertain whether uncomplicated diverticulosis ever gave rise to symptoms. He studied 218 patients and after excluding all those who also had other disorders of the digestive system, he concluded that in only 17 (7·8%) could their symptoms be attributed to their diverticula. Others, including Harold Edwards, were aware of this discrepancy between the presence of symptoms and the absence of diverticulitis, and were struck by the similarity of the symptoms of the 'irritable' or 'spastic' colon syndrome and those of diverticular disease. Edwards (1953) thought that spasticity of the colon might lead on to diverticulosis but, despite many years' observation, failed to establish any causal relationship between the two conditions.

This unsatisfactory state of affairs changed in 1963, when Morson examined sigmoid colons that had been resected at St. Mark's Hospital for the relief of recurrent attacks of severe pain which had been diagnosed as being due to diverticulitis. He found that in only one third of them was there histological evidence of sufficient inflammation to account for the symptoms that had merited major surgery. In some specimens, only the muscle thickening that is so characteristic of the disease was present but *no diverticula could be found*. Thus, the muscle abnormality not only precedes the appearance of diverticula but of itself is capable of causing symptoms of sufficient severity to warrant surgery even when no diverticula are present.

Painter (1964) showed that excessive segmentation of the colon in response to certain stimuli could lead to its lumen being occluded intermittently and later suggested that the colic of so-called diverticulitis is the result of temporary functional obstruction of the colon brought about by segmentation and that this pain is muscular in origin as it waxed and waned with a rapidity that is incompatible with the onset and resolution of an underlying inflammatory process (Painter, 1968). Thus, the pain of uncomplicated diverticular disease owes its origin to a mechanism that is similar to that which causes bladder pain in acute retention of urine. In the former case, the 'little bladders' into which the colon is divided by segmentation, have their outflows obstructed at both ends while, in the latter case, obstruction of the bladder neck results in severe pain even in the absence of any infection.

Obviously, less segmentation will be required if the colon has to cope with soft bulky contents as these can be moved with less effort than would be necessary to shift a viscous faecal stream. Hence, the transportation of soft bulky stools through the sigmoid is less likely to produce colic. Painter, Almeida and Colebourne (1972) made use of this fact when they gave a high fibre diet to 70 patients with uncomplicated diverticular disease. The addition of unprocessed bran to their diet rendered the stools soft and easy to pass and relieved over 85% of their presenting symptoms. Eleven patients who had recurrent severe colic, which would have led to partial colectomy, were made comfortable with bran. This shows that their pain was not due to their diverticula which remained *in situ*.

Furthermore, bran relieved such 'upper intestinal' symptoms as nausea, heartburn, flatulence and distension. Obviously, these symptoms are not due to the presence of diverticula and cannot with any confidence be claimed to be of colonic origin. Therefore, Painter and his colleagues (1972) argued that if a fibre-deficient diet can damage the colonic wall to such an extent as to produce diverticula, it is extremely unlikely that this is the only part of the gut to be adversely affected by our modern diet. They suggested that many of the symptoms that are associated with diverticulosis originate in other parts of the gut which also have not yet adapted to our modern fibre-deficient diet and whose motility is altered by it.

Their concept that the whole of the alimentary tract has to struggle with a low fibre diet would explain not only why 'upper intestinal' symptoms are so commonly associated with diverticular disease, but also how the simple addition of bran to the diet relieves symptoms which appear to arise at different levels of the gastrointestinal tract.

THE CURRENT CLASSIFICATION OF THE MANIFESTATIONS OF DIVERTICULAR DISEASE

These recent advances in the understanding of colonic pathology and physiology have led to the abandonment of the traditional division of the disease into 'diverticulosis' and 'diverticulitis'. Hence the new name. 'Diverticular Disease of the Colon' has been accepted because it has the advantage of shifting attention away from the mucosal herniations and towards the colonic musculature which produces both the diverticula and some of the symptoms that are so often associated with them.

Diverticular disease may be said to be 'uncomplicated' when diverticula are not inflamed and to be 'complicated' if true diverticulitis and its sequelae supervene. The various ways in which the disease may show itself and their relationship to one another are shown diagramatically in Fig. 59. This scheme assumes, perhaps incorrectly, that haemorrhage from diverticula always follows infection and it differs from previous classifications in that it recognizes painful diverticular disease, in which the uninflamed colonic muscle gives rise to colic. This was formerly classified as 'diverticulitis', a term which is now reserved for those manifestations of the disease which are secondary to infection and for which treatment is mainly surgical.

THE PROGNOSIS OF DIVERTICULAR DISEASE

The risk of complications developing in patients with diverticular disease is obviously of the greatest importance as it is only against the background of the natural history of any disease that the efficacy of either medical or surgical treatment can be evaluated. Unfortunately, both the prevalence of the disease

DIVERTICULAR DISEASE OF THE COLON

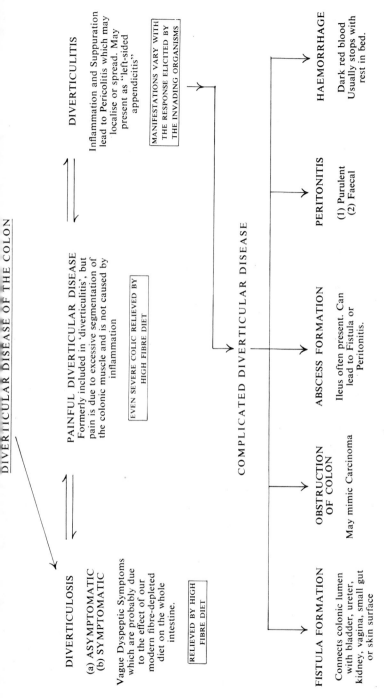

DIVERTICULOSIS

(a) ASYMPTOMATIC
(b) SYMPTOMATIC

Vague Dyspeptic Symptoms which are probably due to the effect of our modern fibre-depleted diet on the whole intestine.

RELIEVED BY HIGH FIBRE DIET

PAINFUL DIVERTICULAR DISEASE
Formerly included in 'diverticulitis', but pain is due to excessive segmentation of the colonic muscle and is not caused by inflammation

EVEN SEVERE COLIC RELIEVED BY HIGH FIBRE DIET

DIVERTICULITIS

Inflammation and Suppuration lead to Pericolitis which may localise or spread. May present as "left-sided appendicitis"

MANIFESTATIONS VARY WITH THE RESPONSE ELICITED BY THE INVADING ORGANISMS

COMPLICATED DIVERTICULAR DISEASE

FISTULA FORMATION

Connects colonic lumen with bladder, ureter, kidney, vagina, small gut or skin surface

OBSTRUCTION OF COLON

May mimic Carcinoma

ABSCESS FORMATION

Ileus often present. Can lead to Fistula or Peritonitis.

PERITONITIS

(1) Purulent
(2) Faecal

HAEMORRHAGE

Dark red blood Usually stops with rest in bed.

Fig. 59. A classification of the manifestations of diverticular disease.

process is changing and the terminology used to describe its various complications has varied over the years, so that the chances of those who have the disease suffering from chronic ill health or requiring surgery for the relief of complications are not known precisely. The few long term studies that have been made are not strictly comparable but they do show that, even in patients attending hospital, the disease usually runs a benign course, but that a significant minority of patients suffer from troublesome symptoms while a few are stricken by the dangerous complications of diverticulitis.

(a) The Extent of Involvement of the Colon

It would be expected that the extent to which the colon is beset with diverticula would affect the chances of diverticulitis supervening; the more the diverticula, the more likely that one of them might become infected. However, this is not so in practice because over 95% of diverticulitis originates in the sigmoid colon. Hence, it is the presence of sigmoid diverticula that sets the stage for complications, and it is usually that part of the sigmoid whose muscle is thickened that is the site of election of diverticulitis. Apart from those in the caecum, diverticula in the proximal colon seldom cause trouble; for some yet unrecognized reason, this is not true of Hawaiian citizens of Japanese stock who usually suffer from diverticulitis of the right half of the colon. For example, Boles and Jordan (1958) followed the progress of 294 patients for a minimum of ten and up to 30 years; no less than one third of them had diverticula scattered throughout their colons and yet, although 176 (40%) of them had at least one attack of diverticulitis, only 73 had complicated diverticular disease. This is because the prognosis with respect to the onset of inflammatory disease is determined by the sigmoid diverticula and the presence of multiple diverticula elsewhere in the colon do not increase the risk of complications significantly (Bolt, 1973).

(b) Does Diverticulosis Spread Round the Colon?

It is generally accepted that the number of diverticula tend to increase with the passing of time and that the disease spreads so as to involve more of the colon (Henderson, 1944). This was the experience of Boles and Jordan in their long follow-up but Parks (1969) observed this happening in only a few patients; he made a retrospective study of the fate of 455 patients with diverticular disease, all of whom had symptoms of sufficient severity to require admission to the Royal Victoria Hospital, Belfast, between 1951 and 1965. Where serial barium enemas were available, they showed that diverticula become established in certain segments and that they tended to progress and distort those segments further rather than to spread along the bowel. This local enlargement of a diverticulum is what would be expected of any hernia but the tendency which he reported of the disease to remain localized to its original segments needs further investigation. Even in Park's series, older patients had more diverticula and he also pointed out that resection of the sigmoid did not prevent diverticula appearing in the proximal colon, whose segments had been normal hitherto. These observations both suggest that more of the colon becomes involved by the disease as the years go by.

The matter is not merely one of academic interest. In recent years, more patients under the age of 50 have been treated by partial colectomy for the relief and prevention of symptoms and so the natural history of the progression of diverticulosis is important. It may be that some of their younger patients will require a further resection later in life if they continue to be subjected to the factors that caused the disease in the first place.

(c) The Incidence of Diverticulitis

The criteria used to diagnose diverticulitis have varied over the years and from observer to observer. Furthermore, most series were studied in retrospect and were selected from those attending hospital clinics, private consulting rooms or from those admitted for treatment, all of which tend to exaggerate the chances of diverticula becoming inflamed. For example, Brown and Marcley (1937), reviewing the progress of 527 patients, classified 220 as having diverticulosis and reported that 277 had diverticulitis treated medically while 99 (16·5%) were treated surgically. One still wonders how many of those who were treated medically had true inflammatory diverticulitis, especially as other observers of this era, including Bargen, Mayo, Oschner and Rankin all placed the incidence of diverticulitis at between 12% and 17%. In a small series, Willard and Bockus (1936) reported that 16 out of 72 (22%) suffered an attack of diverticulitis double the incidence reported by Feldman and Morrison (1949).

At the Lahey Clinic, Boles and Jordan (1958) studied 294 patients who had been observed for a minimum of ten years and up to 30 years with an average of 15 years. The average age was 55 years, but 12 of them were first seen when in their thirties and two when only in their twenties. Complications occurred in 119 (40%) of them; 73 (24·8%) had diverticulitis, 16 (5·4%) haemorrhage, 15 (5·1%) obstruction and 15 (5·1%) perforation or fistula. The benign course of the disease is apparent as only 16 were treated surgically. In another large retrospective series Horner (1958) studied 503 patients who had under observation for a minimum of one year up to 18 years; 85 had one or more episodes of diverticulitis, diagnosed by strict standards, while another 65 were considered to have inflamed diverticula on clinical grounds. This gives an incidence of between 17% and 30% and Horner suggested that a slight difference in the clinical picture might account for the varying prevalence of diverticulitis reported in the literature.

For practical purposes, the estimate of Berman and Kirsner (1972) that about a quarter of those known to have diverticulosis suffer from diverticulitis may be accepted, but this figure would be certainly too high if it were applied to that portion of the population who have undiagnosed diverticula.

(d) The Prognosis following Medical and Surgical Treatment

When the mild forms of the disease, which are treated as outpatients, are studied, the prognosis is very good. Even in the days of the low residue diet and antispasmodics, only 16 of 294 such patients came to surgery (Boles and Jordan, 1958), while of 503 patients in another series, 85 had attacks of diverticulitis but only two were treated surgically (Horner, 1958).

The picture was different when severe forms of diverticular disease, each of which needed treatment in hospital, were considered. Two thirds of 455 patients admitted to a Belfast hospital for treatment of diverticular disease were treated initially by medical means. Of these, no less than one in four had to be readmitted at a later date while 6·3% required a third admission. In the interval between these episodes only 25% were free of symptoms; most were treated by a low residue diet although bulk formers began to come into favour towards the end of the period (1951–1965) that was studied (Parks, 1969; Parks and Connell, 1970).

The clinical state of the 297 medically treated patients was assessed. Five had died from diverticular disease and 81 from other causes and some were not traced. This left 209 patients who had been medically treated and only 122 (58%) were symptom-free; this left 88 patients with symptoms of which 11 (5·3%) were severe (Parks and Connell, 1970). In the same series, 158 of the 455 patients were treated surgically during one or other of their admissions to hospital with 17 deaths, a mortality of 10·7%. Twelve died in their first attack of diverticulitis and nine of them had suffered from symptoms for less than one month. Twenty of the 158 came to operation because of recurrent attacks of diverticulitis that failed to respond to medical management. 107 of the 158 were alive and available for assessment which revealed that no less than 35 (32·7%) were still complaining of symptoms and these included those who had been subjected to resection. A three-stage procedure had been carried out in 25 patients of whom six still had mild symptoms, while 25 had been treated by a one-stage resection and, of these, eight had mild complaints and one still suffered from severe symptoms. Thus, even resection, the last shot in the surgical locker, failed to relieve symptoms in 15 out of 50 patients, an incidence of 30% (Parks, 1969; Parks and Connell, 1970).

This is very similar to the experience of Bolt and Hughes (1966) who reviewed 100 patients with diverticulitis who had undergone laparotomy between five and 15 years previously. Of those who underwent resection 59% remained symptom-free compared with 58% in those who were not treated by resection. They noticed one important difference in these two groups of treated patients. Although both symptoms and recurrent episodes of diverticulitis were mild in the majority of cases, in about 15% of those who had not undergone resection, the disease progressed until either resection was performed or the patient was seriously disabled. In most of the hundred patients who initially had serious complications or fistula, the disease tended to 'burn itself out' with only one late death attributable to the disease (Bolt, 1973).

This difference in the natural history of these two groups is of great importance when the question of prophylactic resection is being considered. There has been a swing towards this in the last 15 years and no less than 70% of patients diagnosed as having diverticulitis at the Lahey Clinic undergo resection to prevent later complications (Colcock, 1971). Brown and Toomey (1960) took the view that earlier surgery would prevent recurrent attacks of diverticulitis. No doubt they were influenced by the fact that 81 of 258 (31%) of their patients had more than one attack of diverticulitis at intervals ranging from one month to ten years. Obviously, it would be a great help to be able to identify the group of patients who are prone to future serious attacks of diverticulitis. At the present it would seem that those with this bad prognosis have a history of weeks or months of increasing symptoms which culminate in an acute episode that requires admission to hospital whereas, in those with a more favourable prognosis, the acute episode occurs almost without warning. The progressive type of the disease has a partially unfavourable prognosis in younger patients but others who have one attack of diverticulitis are unlikely to suffer from another attack. Hence, one acute episode of inflammation is not neces-sarily an indication for resection (Bolt and Hughes, 1966; Parks, 1970; Bolt, 1973).

(e) Prognosis in the Elderly

Diverticulosis becomes commoner with age and, consequently, it affects the elderly who are the very people who also are afflicted by the degenerative diseases of civilization. These in-clude cardiovascular disease, obesity, urinary infection, hiatus hernia, gall-stones and diabetes (Fagin, 1955; Boles and Jordan, 1958; Kyle, 1968; Schowengerdt *et al.*, 1969; Painter *et al.*, 1972). At the age of 70, patients usually show signs of mental or physical deterioration and many of them will not withstand major surgery without a mortality that is unacceptable in a benign con-dition (Bolt, 1960). Furthermore, unless diverticulitis causes complications that threaten life, surgery should be limited to what the patient will stand because often they have only a little while to live even in the absence of diverticular disease. Kyle (1968) found that no less than one third of 206 patients at Aber-deen had died of other diseases at the end of five years. The com-monest causes of death were cardiovascular or cerebrovascular accidents, which was not surprising in view of the fact that one third had evidence of circulatory disease when first they were seen. Hence, although the prognosis of diverticulitis improves with age due to the tendency of the disease to 'burn itself out', the expectancy of life of patients in this age group is decreased considerably by those degenerative diseases which epidemiologically and historically accompany diverticulosis. Consequently, conservative treatment and palliative should be used whenever possible as these elderly patients will not withstand major surgery with an acceptable mortality (Bolt, 1960). As Kyle (1968) remarked, many of these elderly patients with diverticulitis are in as great a need of a good physician as they are of a surgeon.

(f) The Prognosis of Diverticular Disease—A Personal View

The pattern of the natural history of the disease is far from clear, partly because it is changing and partly because the few long term studies have been made on material that has been selected by differing means.

However, it is certain that diverticulosis is affecting younger people and that diverticulitis is becoming commoner under the age of 50. Moreover, it is among these younger patients that those with recurrent severe symptoms and with a bad prognosis are to be found. Is it not possible that this group of patients is suffering from the results of a lifetime of eating a more refined diet than did their parents? This would account for the earlier appearance of diverticulosis and also for this tendency of severe complications to occur in early middle life.

The fact that emerges clearly is that neither medical treatment nor the intervention of the surgeon can guarantee to relieve symptoms in more than 70% of cases. Almost 30% of treated patients continue to suffer from symptoms, which are usually mild but in a small percentage they are still severe enough to make life a misery.

The author believes that there may be a simple reason for these unsatisfactory results. If it is accepted that diverticula result from the ingestion of a fibre-deficient diet for a number of years, then the treatment of attacks of diverticulitis are merely episodes in the history of the disease and if, once these are treated, the abnormal environment of the colon is not changed, then surely the disease would be expected to progress and cause further symptoms? In the studies that have been discussed, patients were treated with the traditional low-residue diet almost throughout these follow-ups (Kyle, 1968; Parks and Connell, 1970) and so not only was the cause of the disease not treated, but the inflamed colon was further insulted by the prescription of a diet even more depleted of fibre. So it is scarcely surprising that the results of both medicine and surgery were so unsatisfactory.

Both Reilly and Daniel prescribe a high fibre diet to those patients on whom they have performed sigmoid myotomy and this combined therapy abolished symptoms in 90% of patients (Daniel, 1969). It is known that myotomy lowers the intra-sigmoid pressures (Smith *et al.*, 1969) but this result is not permanent in those who return to their former diet and the pressures have begun to rise again within two years. However, the reduction in pressure has been maintained for three years so far in patients treated by myotomy who have then changed to a high-fibre diet (Smith, 1973).

The symptoms that accompany uninflamed diverticula can be abolished or relieved in over 85% of patients by the ingestion of a high-fibre/low sugar diet together with millers' bran and these symptoms include severe pain of colonic origin occurring in patients under the age of 50 (Painter, 1972; Painter, Almeida and Colebourne, 1972).

Hence, there is every reason to hope that the prognosis of the disease will alter for the better once we stop treating patients with the disease by giving them the very diet that is responsible for its appearance. Surgery is only an incident in the history of the disease process and so resection should be followed by the taking of adequate cereal fibre. I believe that the general adoption of a high-fibre diet both before diverticulitis has supervened and after surgery will not only change the prognosis of those with the condition, but will improve the results that have so far been reported. A trial of this form of over several years is needed to test this claim.

THE SIZE OF THE CLINICAL PROBLEM
DIVERTICULOSIS

Diverticular disease has become a clinical problem of great magnitude in only 70 years. In 1959 Fox, de Witt and Ponka calculated that by 1975 there would be twenty million Americans over the age of 65. It is known that one third of those over the age of 60 have diverticulosis. They estimated that 20% of them would suffer an attack of diverticulitis and of this million, 15% or 150,000 would need surgical treatment. As long ago as 1930,

Rankin and Brown found that between 14 and 17% of hospital patients with diverticula would suffer from diverticulitis. This figure is probably too high to apply to the population as a whole, and Berman and Kirsner (1972) believe that less than 10% of those with the disease will come to surgery.

Nevertheless, the condition is now so common that if only 10% of diverticulosis patients suffer one attack of diverticulitis and only one in ten of these comes to operation, the problem is great. Furthermore, the complications of the disorder carry a great morbidity and those with uncomplicated diverticulosis have frequently suffered from indigestion and abdominal discomfort for many years before seeking advice. Consequently, although the exact prevalence of diverticula and the incidence of complications are both unknown, one thing is certain, namely, that this benign condition is responsible for a vast amount of chronic ill health among the general population, to say nothing of the mortality and morbidity which attends its dramatic and more publicized complications.

The present situation will get worse if the intake of refined carbohydrates continues to increase or even if it remains the same. Diverticula are being demonstrated ever earlier in life and the disease is no longer confined to 'old and corpulent subjects'. The experience of the last 70 years suggests that if we, as a nation, continue to rely on the processed products of those who purvey flour and foodstuffs for profit, diverticular disease will become an even bigger clinical problem as younger and younger people are affected by our modern fibre-deficient diet.

Chapter 13

Uncomplicated Diverticular Disease

DIVERTICULOSIS

Diverticulosis may be *asymptomatic* as its name suggests. It is certain that the majority of those with the condition have never sought advice regarding their diverticula because they are unaware of their presence. Both the single diverticulum and collections of massed diverticula may give rise to no symptoms. They may be discovered incidentally during a routine radiological examination of the alimentary tract or be found by palpation at operation. However, despite its original definition, diverticulosis is *symptomatic* in more than half of those who are known to have the condition (Berman and Kirsner, 1972).

(a) Symptoms

The disease is associated with vague dyspeptic symptoms which include anorexia, flatulence, nausea, belching, a sensation of abdominal distension and fullness which may be relieved by the passage of faeces or flatus. Flatulence and distension are common symptoms which affect between 25% and 66% of patients (Spriggs and Marxer, 1925; Todd, 1955). These symptoms are not specific as they are common to other disorders of the alimentary tract and so diverticulosis is difficult to differentiate on clinical grounds from hiatus hernia, peptic ulcer, carcinoma of the stomach, biliary disease, recurrent appendicitis and other colonic disorders. Some patients complain of aching or heaviness in the lower abdomen, symptoms common in constipation and in some gynaecological conditions.

The clinical diagnosis of diverticulosis is made more difficult by the fact that all these disorders are common in the Western nations who eat a fibre-deficient diet and that, consequently, these other conditions are found frequently together with diverticulosis in the same patient (Fagin, 1955; Boles and Jordan, 1958; Kyle, 1968; Painter *et al.*, 1972). This makes it difficult, if not impossible, to attribute any particular symptoms to the diverticula.

(b) The Bowel Habit in Diverticulosis

It was once thought that diverticula were caused by constipation. This idea was abandoned when the bowel habits of those with diverticulosis were compared with those of their fellow citizens. Diverticula were found in patients who were regular and in some who passed stools frequently. Edwards (1939) said that the bowel habit in the disease was variable and that some patients might be alternately costive or loose. It must be remembered that constipation is defined differently by different authors and that the word means one thing in this country and quite another to the rural African who considers himself unwell if he only defaecates once a day. In those countries where diverticulosis has become common, small stiff stools pass through the colon slowly and are often voided with an effort, whereas in the developing countries, where the disease is extremely rare, bulky soft faeces are passed more than once a day without an effort (Burkitt, Walker and Painter, 1972 and 1974). Hence, it is not surprising that the pattern of the bowel habit differs greatly in the published reports.

A survey of the American and British literature shows that from 14% to 60% of patients with diverticulosis are constipated, 4% to 39% suffer from diarrhoea or pass stools frequently, while from 14% to 54% are said to be regular; in from 3% to 10% of patients the bowel habit alternates between constipation and the passage of loose stools (Spriggs and Marxer, 1925; Oschner and Bargen, 1935; Willard and Bockus, 1936; Brown and Marcley, 1937; Feldman and Morrison, 1949; Horner, 1958; Havia, 1971; Painter, Almeida and Colebourne, 1972).

On average, more than one half of patients pass at least one motion a day; some may defaecate twelve times a day and some only once a week. It is important to question patients as to the bulk and consistency of their stools. It is easy to interpret a history of several bowel actions a day as meaning that the patient is not constipated and even to assume that he passes soft or loose stools. Closer enquiry will often reveal that the patient never feels that his rectum empties completely and that he or she goes to the lavatory several times a day but only passes a small piece of hard faeces at each sitting. These often weigh less than 40 grams, and such 'sheep droppings' are voided only after considerable straining. It is these patients who often complain that their rectum is never empty. In 70 patients with symptomatic diverticulosis, six patients were distressed by this symptom to the extent that they were conscious of a full rectum throughout the day; all six were relieved by a high fibre diet with added bran (Painter *et al.*, 1972).

Some patients who are constipated suffer from attacks of diarrhoea which may be accompanied by the passage of mucus and sometimes blood. These episodes occur spontaneously or follow the taking of laxatives. This pattern of bowel behaviour is similar to that seen in 'mucous colitis', a variety of constipation described by a previous generation of physicians, and which probably results from hard scyballa irritating the lining of the colon and producing catarrh.

The bowel habit may be altered by purgatives and up to two thirds of patients with the disease have taken some form of laxative habitually or intermittently. The pattern of bowel behaviour may also change suddenly if the colonic lumen is narrowed by recurrent diverticulitis or by a co-existing neoplasm.

Any alteration in the bowel habit or the passage of blood or mucus in the stools must be investigated thoroughly to exclude the presence of a carcinoma. This is also true of patients who are already known to have diverticulosis. Diverticular disease and cancer of the large bowel have the same epidemiology and so it is not surprising that they may occur together in the same patient. This fact must always be borne in mind.

(c) The Diagnosis and Investigation of Diverticulosis

(i) *History*

The diagnosis is suspected from the history. The symptoms listed above should always bring the diagnosis to mind in patients over the age of 40. At the age of 60, the diagnosis will be right in this country in one of every three patients purely on statistical grounds. It should be remembered also that diverticula are being found in younger people, being not uncommon in those below the age of 40 and are even appearing in the third decade of life.

Diverticula may co-exist with any of the other diseases of the alimentary tract that have become common in the Western nations (Cleave, Campbell and Painter, 1969). The so-called 'Saint's Triad' described by Muller (1948) is only one example of how a combination of these 'diseases of civilization' may be found together in the same patient. Consequently, the possible presence of diverticulosis should not be forgotten when some abnormality of the upper intestinal tract has been demonstrated; the lower bowel should be examined radiographically as well, especially in older patients.

(ii) *Clinical Examination*

Usually, all that the clinical examination reveals is that the pelvic colon is palpable and can be rolled under the examining fingers. Sometimes the colon is contracted and tender and resembles a rigid rubber hose having a diameter of about one and a half inches. This is not diagnostic of diverticulosis because, except in obese patients, this part of the colon can be felt in the majority of people in this country whether they have diverticula or not and, also, because the colon feels the same in the so-called 'irritable colon syndrome'.

Digital examination of the rectum must always be carried out. This will exclude stenosis of the anus and rectal carcinoma and will reveal the consistency of any faeces that are present in the rectum. If hard pellets of faeces are felt in the rectum of a patient who says he has six bowel actions a day it is at once obvious that he does not suffer from diarrhoea but that he is constipated and probably voids hard pieces of faeces several times a day. The presence of blood or mucus on the glove must never be attributed to diverticulosis even when the disease is already known to be present. The state of the anal mucosa and the presence or absence of piles are then assessed with a proctoscope. These findings must be followed by a full investigation of the large bowel unless a barium enema and sigmoidoscopy have been performed in the very recent past.

(iii) *Sigmoidoscopy*

Sigmoidoscopy is essential to exclude the presence of other diseases, especially malignant growths of the rectum and lower sigmoid colon. The author sigmoidoscopes his patients at their first visit immediately after the clinical examination and in the knee-elbow position if this is possible. The mucosa is then unaffected by previous washouts and while a small amount of faeces may be present in the rectum these can usually be circumnavigated with the instrument so that a good view is obtained. If the rectum is so loaded with faeces that this is impossible, or any blood or mucus of unexplained origin is seen, then the patient is admitted as soon as possible for examination after a thorough preparation to make sure that a carcinoma is not responsible for these abnormalities.

Sigmoidoscopy is rarely helpful in diagnosing diverticula whose mouths are not easily seen, although Jackman and Buie (1943) managed to see these in 35 out of 242 patients with the disease. An acute angle at about 15 cm. from the anal margin is consistent with the diagnosis of diverticulosis. It may be impossible to pass the instrument beyond this point, especially if previous attacks of diverticulitis have rendered the sigmoid rigid or adherent to neighbouring structures or have narrowed its lumen. The sigmoid colon may be mobile but narrowed by semi-lunar folds which do not pass right round the bowel but which project from each side towards each other so as to divide the colon into saccules. These folds may yield to the insufflation of air or give way with gentle pressure as the sigmoidoscope is gently but firmly advanced. This state of affairs is not diagnostic of the condition as it is common to the so-called 'spastic' colon and may be seen even when no diverticula can be demonstrated (Buie, 1939; Jackman and Buie, 1943).

(iv) *Barium Enema Examination of the Colon*

Diverticulosis must be diagnosed by barium enema, preferably of the double contrast type which is more likely to demonstrate any other abnormalities such as growths which may exist concurrently with diverticulosis. The radiology of diverticular disease is discussed by Dr Kreel in Chapter 4. It must be stressed that if diverticula are discovered incidentally by a barium meal that has been followed through the gut, the colon must be examined by a barium enema as well not only to assess the extent of the disease process but also to exclude the presence of a carcinoma.

Similarly, when diverticula have been found by a barium enema, they must not be blamed for symptoms until the rest of the alimentary canal has been searched for evidence of the other diseases that are so often associated with diverticulosis. Only in the absence of other disorders can either dyspeptic symptoms, abdominal discomfort or symptoms referable to the large bowel be attributed to diverticulosis. Furthermore, it should be remembered that uninflamed diverticula are merely *associated* with these symptoms which, like them, are caused by disordered motility of the bowels' musculature.

(v) *Other Investigations*

A full blood count may reveal that the patient is anaemic. This may be due to bleeding from diverticula or another colonic lesion. The stools should be examined for occult blood. The urine should be cultured as urinary infection in diverticulosis may herald the development of a vesico-colic fistula. It is important to exclude the presence of diabetes mellitus as this is often associated with diverticular disease (Schowengerdt *et al.*, 1969).

(d) The Treatment of Diverticulosis

Once diverticula have been demonstrated and the presence of colonic cancer has been ruled out, a decision must be made as to whether the patient's symptoms merit treatment. Some doctors do not tell the patient of the presence of asymptomatic diverticula lest they worry unduly. This attitude is almost always wrong. Everyone fears the unknown more than the known and patients will co-operate with the doctor who takes them into his confidence. This is essential. The taking of a high-fibre diet requires thought and care by the patient and in my experience patients cease to worry once the nature of diverticulosis and its relation to diet is explained to them. This is best done with the aid of a simple diagram such as is shown in Chapter 21 ; this can be sketched while describing the anatomy of the colon and of diverticula to the patient.

Once patients understand that they have a benign condition, that will respond to simple dietary changes, they take an intelligent interest in what they eat, often to the benefit of their family, their friends and their work-mates. They are told to report at once if any blood or mucus is passed with their stools or if their bowel habit changes. This helps to ensure that obstruction of the colon due to carcinoma of the colon or diverticulitis is discovered early. It is particularly important that any urinary symptoms are reported at once as they may herald the formation of a vesico-colic fistula.

The hallowed regimen of a low residue diet and liquid paraffin has been abandoned. The former is contra-indicated because it is the cause of the disease and the prolonged use of liquid paraffin (mineral oil) may cause vitamin deficiency (Black, 1953; Becker, 1954), faecal incontinence (Curtis and Kline, 1939) or lipoid pneumonia (Forbes and Bradley, 1958). The author has assisted at a lobectomy performed for a suspected carcinoma of the lung which proved to be a 'paraffinoma'.

The modern treatment of the disease should ensure that the bowels are kept open easily and the stools are soft, bulky and passed without straining. If no significant effort is needed to void the motions it is reasonable to suppose that they have been propelled through the colon with the minimum of segmentation and pressure production. This is achieved by the use of unprocessed millers' bran to ensure that the diet has a high fibre content and the reduction of the intake of refined sugar. The high fibre diet is described in Chapter 21. Those who do not tolerate bran should be given Sterculia in the form of Normacol Standard or Normacol Special; this is known as Movicol in the United States of America. This is the best alternative to bran as it has not been known to clump and cause obstruction and neither does it impart a greasy texture to the stools; these disadvantages have been reported with other bulk formers.

Purgatives, enemas and colonic lavage should be avoided. Obese patients should reduce weight as this will render any subsequent surgery safer.

Milk is contraindicated in some patients, especially in its raw state. Mucus and blood may be passed per rectum during episodes of diarrhoea in susceptible patients even after half a cupful of milk. Corry (1963) advised all his patients to manage without milk for two weeks and said this gave relief to 12 out of 120 patients. One of the author's patients, a lady of 62 took milk before retiring to bed and this was followed by the passage of five loose motions in the next two hours. This stopped when she gave up milk. After sigmoidectomy she could drink milk freely without any ill effects. The reason for this effect of milk is not yet known.

A high fibre diet will abolish or relieve over 85% of the symptoms of the disease once the correct daily dosage of bran has been ascertained by the patient. It will cure constipation so that the need for laxatives is minimal (Dimock, 1936). However, it will not prevent future attacks of painful diverticular disease nor attacks of diverticulitis (Painter, Almeida and Colebourne, 1972). A long term trial conducted over many years will be required before it is known whether the addition of cereal fibre to the diet will alter the prognosis in diverticular disease. In the meantime, there is plenty of clinical evidence that it is of great benefit.

Anticholinergic drugs have been used in an attempt to reduce the 'spasm' or alter the motility of the colon. Probanthine tablets 15 mg. three times a day with two tablets (30 mg.) given at night are given at first and later increased until the patient complains of dryness of the mouth and mucous membranes. There is no evidence that this dosage of probanthine or any other antispasmodic are of any benefit. Some clinicians use Merbentyl 10 mg. three times a day and 20 mg. at night for painful diverticula disease in the hope that it will relieve pain (Eastwood, personal communication, 1973). Antispasmodics have unpleasant side effects when given in large doses. They may make the mucous membranes dry and their use has been followed by acute retention of urine. The author has never been convinced that oral antispasmodics are helpful and has not prescribed them since he began to use bran eight years ago.

When patients have been investigated fully and their symptoms have been relieved by these simple dietary changes, they are returned to the care of their family doctor. They should continue to eat a high fibre diet for life and should report to their doctor if any of their old symptoms recur or any new ones appear. They are told to seek advice if they pass blood or mucus per rectum or if they notice any urinary symptoms. Theoretically, their colon should be examined at intervals but the logistics of such an exercise make this impracticable. Hence the need to explain to patients the nature of their condition and to ensure that they know which of these symptoms should be taken seriously. It is only with the patients' co-operation that complications will be detected early in their development.

PAINFUL DIVERTICULAR DISEASE

Pain in the left iliac fossa or in the lower abdomen may be felt by patients with diverticular disease even when there is no evidence that their diverticula are inflamed. In the past this was attributed incorrectly to 'diverticulitis' although some authors considered that mild examples of the condition were manifestations of an 'irritable' or 'spastic' colon. It is now known that these symptoms ranging from discomfort to severe colic are caused by excessive segmentation of the sigmoid causing intermittent functional obstruction. The pain is of muscular origin because, like labour pains, or the colic of obstruction, it waxes and wanes with a rapidity that is incompatible with the development and resolution of an inflammatory process (Painter, 1968).

(a) Symptoms

The symptoms are those of diverticulosis overshadowed by recurrent episodes of pain. This pain is often remittent rather than intermittent as a dull ache often persists between the recurrent attacks of colic. This pain is described as 'cramping' or 'colicky' and women may remark that 'it is like little labour pains' while pointing to their left lower abdomen. The intensity of the pain may vary from an annoying ache, similar to that felt in the 'irritable colon syndrome', to colic that may be so severe that it is attributed erroneously to the passing of a ureteric calculus (Painter, Almeida & Colebourne, 1972). Such pain will cause the patient to go to bed, often with a hot water bottle. Food may aggravate the pain, presumably this is due to the 'gastro-colic reflex'. Pain may be felt in the right iliac fossa if the colon crosses the mid-line. Both the colic and any sensation of distension may be relieved by the passage of wind or faeces but sometimes defaecation is followed by an exacerbation of the colic.

The bowel habit varies; either constipation or diarrhoea may accompany these episodes of pain. The passage of blood or mucus must be investigated as soon as the acute attack has subsided to exclude the presence of a neoplasm and must never be attributed to the diverticula until this has been done.

(b) History

There may be no history of former symptoms because the first attack of pain may occur without warning in a previously healthy patient (Parks, 1969). On the other hand, the patient may have suffered recurrent episodes of pain and be known to have diverticulosis. Some patients have been diagnosed as having a spastic colon, when, in fact, their sigmoid probably was in the 'prediverticular state'. The history may suggest obstruction from adhesions or left renal colic, but in most patients, the history points to some disorder of the colon.

(c) Clinical Examination

Although the patient may be in pain, there is no evidence of a constitutional upset such as accompanies appendicitis, diverticulitis or peritonitis. Palpation of the abdomen reveals a tender contracted pelvic colon but no evidence of local peritonitis. Once the patient has been persuaded to relax and this may take time, the course of the pelvic colon can be defined by gentle but firm palpation, except in obese patients. Although the contracted colon is tender, as in the irritable colon syndrome, it can be defined with the examining fingers. This is in contrast to acute diverticulitis in which pericolitis and the involvement of adjacent serosal surfaces soon leads to reflex guarding. Even when peritonitis is still localized, the abdominal muscles will not relax and the left iliac fossa is diffusely tender and the colon cannot be defined as in painful diverticular disease.

Rectal examination is not diagnostic and sigmoidoscopy is seldom helpful, the bowel often being angled above the rectosigmoid junction and its lumen so contracted that any attempt to advance the instrument results in pain. If diverticulitis has supervened, pain will be felt if either the finger or the sigmoidoscope disturbs the inflamed tissues and sigmoidoscopy should then be delayed until the attack has subsided.

(d) Investigations

A full blood count will show that the white count and sedimentation rate are both normal. The urine is cultured and the stools examined for occult blood. A barium enema should not be performed until all symptoms have subsided as perforation may follow any enema given during an acute episode of pain. The colon must be examined radiographically after the patient has recovered unless it has been examined in this way in the recent past.

(e) Diagnosis

The diagnosis is made from the history and examination together with the absence of any clinical or laboratory evidence of true inflammatory diverticulitis. This applies only to patients who are known to have diverticulosis. If the colon has not been examined radiologically before the attack, the diagnosis remains provisional until the presence of diverticula has been demonstrated.

The differential diagnosis includes other causes of abdominal colic, notably left renal colic and of course diverticulitis and pericolitis.

(f) Treatment

The patient should rest and in a severe attack should be confined to bed. The presence of diverticulitis, pericolitis and peritonitis must be excluded by repeated examination and by the absence of fever and any change in the white cell count. At any time, and with little warning, the clinical picture may change. Diverticulitis may develop or a mucosal pouch may perforate. The onset of these complications may be very sudden and so if there is any doubt as to the diagnosis, any deterioration in the patient's condition or any increase in the severity of the pain, the patient should be admitted immediately to hospital. In this country, where hospitals are close at hand, the general practitioner would be well advised to seek the opinion of a surgeon at a domiciliary visit or to arrange for the patient's admission so that his condition can be observed continuously. This is impossible in the patient's home unless a private nurse is available.

When the diagnosis is certain, a light diet with plenty of fluids is given together with a bulk former. The author gives miller's bran but this may increase the feeling of distension, in which case sterculia in the form of Normacol or Normacol Standard (Movicol in the U.S.A.), is given to ensure that the sigmoid will not have to struggle with a viscous faecal stream once its present contents have been evacuated. During convalescence, the sterculia can be replaced by bran in most cases.

Pain is relieved by pethidine (demerol) given intramuscularly. This is the analgesic of choice. While it exerts its central effect, this drug will relax the bowel's smooth muscle. *Morphine is contra-indicated* because it raises the intracolonic pressures by promoting segmentation of the sigmoid and so favours the perforation of diverticula. Antispasmodics are claimed to be helpful, but seem to have a negligible effect when given by mouth.

There is no doubt that probanthone given intramuscularly or intravenously will relax the colon, sometimes with the relief of pain, but its side effects are unpleasant. It may cause ileus and a sudden regurgitation of the stomach's contents in patients who are supine in bed; this is not without danger.

Purgatives and enemas must be withheld as these may be followed by perforation. The object is to rest the sigmoid, not to stimulate it. Some patients noticed that milk, particularly in its natural state, exacerbates their symptoms and they should avoid it (Corry, 1963).

(g) Management after an Attack of Painful Diverticular Disease

The attack subsides providing diverticulitis does not develop. The patient is then placed on a high-fibre/low sugar diet. The patient eats wholemeal bread and miller's bran in such a quantity as to render the stools sufficiently soft to allow them to be voided without straining at least once, but preferably twice, a day. The regimen to be followed is the same as that outlined for diverticulosis. This does not guarantee that the patient will not suffer from attacks of painful diverticular disease or diverticulitis in the future but, in the interval, patients are usually symptom free on the high-fibre diet whereas formerly 30% of medically treated patients continued to have symptoms (Painter, Almeida and Colebourne, 1972).

Some patients notice that episodes of pain are precipitated by emotional stress and a small dose of phenobarbitone or a tranquillizer may lessen the frequency and the severity of their symptoms. Some have found that one glass of whisky will allay their anxiety and abolish pain in their left iliac fossa.

The prognosis is good: the majority of patients respond to this simple change in their diet. A few will continue to have pain so frequently that their life becomes intolerable. These should be cured by colectomy or sigmoid myotomy (Painter, 1968).

Chapter 14

Complicated Diverticular Disease: Diverticulitis and Abscess Formation

Diverticular disease may give rise to two complications, inflammation and haemorrhage. Diverticulitis means that one or more diverticula are inflamed and the term is no longer used to describe pain caused by contraction of the colonic musculature. This is referred to as painful diverticular disease (Painter, 1968) or spastic colon diverticulosis (Fleischner, 1971).

PATHOLOGY

Recent investigators agree that diverticulitis originates in the inflammation of one diverticulum which perforates. Once the serosa covering the thin sac of mucosa has been breached the bacteria which normally inhabit the bowel escape into the peritoneal cavity where an abscess may form. The further progress of this pathological process will depend on the body's response to these invading organisms (Morson, 1963; Fleischner, Ming and Henken, 1964; Fleischner and Ming, 1965). Why the diverticulum becomes inflamed by bacteria which are normally resident in the colonic lumen is not known for certain. Mechanical trauma due to inspissated faeces has been suggested as a cause, but it may be that high intracolonic pressures play a part. The colon can generate pressures in excess of 90 mm./Hg which not only distend diverticula but which are far greater than the pressure of the intramural blood vessels of the colon. Consequently, it is possible that the colonic mucosa and that of diverticula may be devitalized by abnormally high intrasigmoid pressures so that it can be invaded by bacterial flora to which it is normally resistant; a similar trigger mechanism may be responsible for acute appendicitis (Painter, 1967; Burkitt, 1971). Diverticular disease and arteriosclerosis are both diseases of civilization which became clinical problems at about the same time. Both have the same geographical distribution and both affect older patients (Trowell, Painter and Burkitt, 1974) and so it would not be surprising if, at some future date, excessive intracolonic pressure and vascular insufficiency were shown to play a part in the causation of acute diverticulitis.

Once a diverticulum has perforated, its infected contents escape into the peritoneal cavity. Often, the perforation is small and it is walled off by adjacent tissues and only a small localized abscess forms which may drain back into the bowel so that the episode of diverticulitis resolves. Such an incident may give rise to a minimum of symptoms.

Alternatively, the inflammation may spread along the colon so that several segments are involved. This *pericolitis* may be accompanied by the formation of one or more localized small abscesses. The inflammation is localized by the adjacent viscera and by the omentum and this results in a varying degree of paralytic ileus and distension of the small bowel. Resolution may follow this stage in the pathological process.

An abscess may cause the colon to become adherent to a neighbouring viscus such as the bladder. If the abscess discharges into this viscus a *fistula* is formed; the commonest variety being a *vesico-colic* fistula, or more correctly a colo-vesical fistula.

Sometimes a pericolic abscess that has been localized will rupture suddenly and without warning. Its contents then spill into the general peritoneal cavity giving rise to *purulent peritonitis*. If the perforation is large and the tissues show but little response against the invading organisms, the perforation will remain open so that not only does the peritoneum become infected but the situation is worsened still further by the outpouring of the contents of the bowel. This dreaded complication is known as *faecal peritonitis*.

Acute diverticulitis and pericolitis may cause temporary obstruction, not only of the small bowel by inducing ileus, but also of the sigmoid colon. This may already have its lumen narrowed by muscle thickening so that inflammatory oedema may narrow it further so that it is obstructed temporarily. Some degree of obstruction was present in two thirds of the 258 cases of diverticulitis that were reviewed by Brown and Toomey (1960).

DIVERTICULITIS, PERICOLITIS AND PERICOLIC ABSCESS

These are part of the same inflammatory process which may progress to fistula formation or to peritonitis. However, if treatment is successful, these latter complications may be avoided.

(c) Symptoms

Diverticulitis causes local peritonitis. Pain is felt which is more constant than that of painful diverticular disease and it lasts until the inflammatory process subsides. This pain may occur suddenly in a previously symptom-free patient or in one who has suffered from episodes of colic in the past. It is felt usually in the left iliac fossa and is accompanied by fever, malaise, anorexia, distension, and a constitutional upset, all of which serve to distinguish it from painful diverticular disease. Obstruction from ileus or oedema of the colon may give rise to colic and distension which is relieved by passing flatus and which may be accompanied by nausea. Tenderness and guarding which is maximal over the affected bowel reveals the presence of local peritonitis; this is felt usually in the left iliac fossa but the condition can be mistaken for appendicitis if the colon curves across the midline.

If the peritonitis is spreading, suprapubic pain with tenderness and guarding in both lower quadrants of the abdomen make the precise diagnosis uncertain. Low backache is common. Botsford and Curtis (1961) reported that 28 out of 100 patients complained of this symptom. Botsford and Zollinger (1969) state that this is a common finding but that it is seldom reported.

The bowel habit varies from constipation to diarrhoea. Vomiting only occurs secondary to ileus caused by the involvement of small gut in the inflammatory process. Blood may be passed per rectum. This is dull red unlike that due to bleeding piles and usually stops with rest in bed, but sometimes massive haemorrhage threatens life. The passing of blood must never be attributed to diverticulosis until the presence of a carcinoma or other colonic disease has been excluded.

CLINICAL EXAMINATION

Except in mild attacks, the patient is ill, in pain and looks toxic. Palpation reveals the presence of local peritonitis; this may be felt only on deep palpation of the sigmoid in mild cases. A careful search is made for any tender mass which indicates the presence of an abscess. A pelvic abscess may only be felt on rectal examination, but guarding and obesity may make it impossible to detect even a large collection of pus, especially if this is high in the pelvis.

The examiner's next problem is to judge whether the inflammatory process is localized or whether it is spreading. Even very experienced surgeons may find this extremely difficult. The nearer the finger tips can approach and define the inflamed colon or abscess, the more likely is it that the infection is localized. This applies *only at the time of examination* as the situation may change suddenly and so repeated examinations must be made at intervals. Hence, the patient is best admitted to hospital for observation in an attack of diverticulitis. The bowel sounds are decreased or absent depending on the degree of ileus.

Failure of the inflammation to localize results in the tenderness becoming more marked and more diffuse. Any mass that has been outlined may enlarge. It is easier to notice these changes if all examinations are carried out by the same observer. The bowel sounds will diminish or disappear if peritonitis is spreading and guarding will progress to rigidity.

Proctoscopy and sigmoidoscopy will allow the state of the rectum to be assessed and the presence of a carcinoma to be excluded. These must be performed gently and only if the patient's condition permits. It is seldom possible to pass the instrument into the sigmoid because of pain and tenderness, or to make a diagnosis by this means.

RADIOGRAPHIC EXAMINATION OF THE COLON

A barium enema is contraindicated in acute diverticulitis as it may be followed by perforation. However, unless one has been performed very recently, a barium enema must be performed as soon as the attack has subsided to make the diagnosis and to detect any narrowing of the colon which may be due to diverticulitis, carcinoma or both conditions being present together. Such an examination may also reveal the presence of Crohn's disease or ulcerative colitis which may co-exist with diverticulosis.

OTHER INVESTIGATIONS

The temperature, pulse, white cell count and sedimentation rate are raised. An erect radiograph of the abdomen will show fluid levels if obstruction is present and gas under the diaphragm if free perforation is present. This examination is only carried out when the condition of the patient allows this manoeuvre. The urine is examined for sugar and cultured. Diabetes is often associated with diverticulitis and urinary infection may be due to a fistula. The stools should be examined for blood.

DIFFERENTIAL DIAGNOSIS

Diverticulitis must be differentiated from appendicitis, salpingitis and other cause of peritonitis; sometimes this may be impossible except at laparotomy. The condition may be mistaken for the irritable colon syndrome, intestinal obstruction, renal colic, endometriosis or other colonic disorders such as Crohn's disease and ulcerative colitis.

The detection of Crohn's disease when it exists with diverticulitis was discussed by Schmidt and his colleagues (1968). In their series of 137 patients with Crohn's disease, no less than 26 had colonic diverticula as well. This dual pathology is seen more in women than men and affects the prognosis profoundly. Sigmoidoscopy revealed an abnormality in 23 of the 26 cases, while 24 of the 26 had either an anal lesion or a recto-vaginal fistula. This examination is most important as radiology may show only diverticula. A pre-operative diagnosis of Crohn's disease is important because seven of 14 patients operated upon who had both diseases developed complications. In three the anastomosis broke down to form an external fistula and three developed recto-vaginal fistula; the wound healed slowly in two and chronic anal fissures and fistulae also occurred. These complications are seldom seen in patients who only have diverticulosis.

The association of diverticulitis and acute ulcerative colitis is fortunately uncommon as it carries a high mortality. One quarter of patients with ulcerative colitis who have passed the age of 60 have colonic diverticula, an incidence that is similar to that found in the rest of the population. Hence, the acute varieties of the two conditions must be expected to co-exist on occasions but, in practice, the 'double' diagnosis is seldom made before laparotomy (Bates and Karminsky, 1974). It has been suggested that ulcerative colitis can involve the mucosal sacs and hence give rise to secondary diverticulitis, but Jalan and his colleagues (1970) found that the mucosal inflammation stopped at the necks of the diverticula.

Diverticulitis may cause a degree of obstruction of the sigmoid and it is possible that this precipitates toxic dilatation of the proximal colon, a complication requiring immediate total colectomy. By contrast, colitis of the distal colon may lead to faecal stasis in the right half of the colon without dilatation, presumably because there is no degree of obstruction (Lennard–Jones *et al.*, 1962).

Bates and Karminsky (1974) suggest that sigmoidoscopy should be repeated in a patient with diverticulitis whose condition suddenly deteriorates. The pre-operative recognition of ulcerative colitis would prevent the wrong operation, namely a local segmental resection for diverticulitis, being performed when it was the colitic component that was threatening life.

TREATMENT

The patient should be nursed in hospital. No solid food is allowed. Fluids may be given orally but, if ileus is present, they must be given intravenously when gastric suction must be instituted and the electrolytes estimated. Some degree of obstruction is seen in up to two thirds of those suffering from diverticulitis. If appendicitis can be excluded with confidence and the inflammatory process is localized, broad spectrum antibiotics are given. These must be given intramuscularly or intravenously if the patient is nauseated and in a dosage sufficient to attain a blood level adequate to combat bacteria that have escaped from the bowel and invaded the tissues. Attempts to sterilize the bowel with non-absorbable antibiotics are pointless, as the colon is accustomed to accommodating its normal inhabitants. Pethidine (demerol) is given to relieve pain because it decreases the motility of the colon and therefore helps to rest it. Morphine is contra-indicated as it has the reverse effect.

Purgatives and enemas must not be given as they disturb the inflamed colon and have been known to cause perforation.

The patient's condition must be watched closely and assessed and examined repeatedly to ensure that an abscess is not enlarging or the peritonitis is not spreading. Conservative treatment may be rewarded by the resolution of the diverticulitis. This is shown by the gradual disappearance of signs and symptoms, the return of the appetite and a steady improvement of the patient's general condition.

After recovery from the attack, the state of the colon must be investigated by barium enema and sigmoidoscopy to exclude co-existing carcinoma, Crohn's disease, ulcerative colitis or any narrowing resulting from diverticulitis. The barium may escape from the bowel and outline a track or an abscess cavity. Any urinary infection should be treated vigorously, while pyelography and cystoscopy will make sure that no nephro-colic, uretero-colic or vesico-colic fistula has formed. A left hydronephrosis may be due to diverticulosis of the sigmoid and yet overshadow the primary disease (Hersh and Schwabe, 1963). Cystoscopy seldom shows the opening of a fistula as usually this is obscured by granulation tissue. This should be biopsied; a negative result does not exclude the presence of cancer. The differential diagnosis of neoplastic and inflammatory narrowing of the colon and fistula formation is discussed elsewhere in this book.

DIVERTICULITIS WITH ABSCESS FORMATION

An abscess may resolve or be so small that it is only identified by the pathologist when examining colons resected following diverticulitis, alternatively it may enlarge. An abscess may still localize even when it is bigger than a clenched fist or presents on rectal examination as a bulge that resembles a foetal head. Abscess formation causes a swinging temperature and a rise in the white cell count. Oedema of the colon and other viscera often cause local ileus so that some degree of obstruction attends two thirds of cases (Brown and Toomey, 1960). While a large abscess may discharge into the bowel and diminish in size, it also may point towards the skin in the left lower abdomen or burst into the bladder or small gut to form a fistula.

Unpleasant though these complications may be, the most

dangerous state of affairs follows the rupture of the wall of a large abscess. A considerable mass of pus and debris is then released without warning into the general peritoneal cavity. The patient, who was thought to be improving, suddenly becomes shocked as peritonitis spreads rapidly.

Conservative treatment of a palpable abscess always carries the very real risk of spreading peritonitis and the high mortality which attends this complication. A false sense of security may be engendered by the use of gastric suction, intravenous therapy, antibiotics and analgesics, all of which tend to mask symptoms. This is especially so in obese patients. Consequently, it is essential to examine the patient at regular intervals so that if there is the slightest suspicion that the abscess is failing to subside, it can be drained without delay. A faecal fistula may follow drainage if the perforation that caused the abscess is still open.

Drainage of the abscess should be achieved by the shortest route, so as to avoid contaminating the general peritoneal cavity. The object is to assist the colon to rest and the natural defences to overcome the infection which is threatening life and not to subject the patient to a long and difficult operation while in a debilitated state. The establishment of a transverse colostomy on the right hand side is simple and adds little to the operation time (McLaren, 1957). This will divert the faecal stream and rest the distal colon. Following this operation, resection of the colon should be delayed for a minimum of four months, and probably for six months, unless the presence of cancer cannot be ruled out. The inflammation will subside in these months making resection easier and the patient's condition will improve making surgery safer. Obesity is a common problem and the patient will have time to shed some fat before this second operation.

The second stage consists of resection of the diseased sigmoid including the recto-sigmoid junction. The colostomy is closed at a third operation after the patency of the anastomosis has been checked radiographically. A colostomy must never be closed without prior resection of the diseased bowel that is distal to it. If this rule is broken, there is a very great risk of recurrent diverticulitis accompanied by worse complications than those which the patient has withstood already. These have often proved fatal. Better to leave a patient with a colostomy than to close it with a permanently damaged and probably narrowed bowel beyond it.

Although this three-stage programme has been proved to be save since Smithwick (1942) used it to revolutionize our approach to diverticular disease, several surgeons have recommended a one stage procedure in which the abscess is drained and the colon together with its perforation are removed at one operation. If successful this saves hospital beds and expense (Noer, 1959; Ponka and Hays, 1972). Alternatively, primary resection may be accompanied by a colostomy to protect the anastomosis so that the patient is cured with two operations (Byrne and Garick, 1971). Between 1945 and 1954, the proportion of patients treated by one-stage resection rose from 9.7% to over 52% in some centres (Waugh and Walt, 1959). No doubt primary resection is the ideal but in my opinion it should be undertaken only by an experienced surgeon under ideal conditions. At the best of times, an anastomosis low in the colon is less reliable than one in the rest of the gut and its safety is further put at risk by the presence of pus, exudate and oedema of the tissues. Furthermore, the mobilization of the left colon, that may be necessary to obtain normal bowel to anastomose to the upper rectum, also serves to open up tissue planes for the spread of infection. Resection is safest when the inflammatory process has settled and when the colon has been defunctioned for six months (Botsford and Zollinger, 1969; Colcock, 1971). The author has abandoned a resection in favour of a colostomy when laparotomy showed that the sigmoid colon and adjacent tissues were still oedematous even after six months, although the operation had been started in the belief that a previous episode of diverticulitis had subsided. Rodkey and Welch (1969) stressed that primary resection in the presence of complications should be used with extreme caution.

In contrast to the proven safety of staged resection, the dehissence of a primary anastomosis is disastrous. Even if the situation is retrieved by prompt intervention, the patient is worse off than before the operation. Botsford, Zollinger and Hicks (1971) reviewed 252 operations for diverticulitis. They found that five anastomotic leaks protected by a colostomy all healed and no patient died and said, 'in marked contrast, four of the five patients with anastomotic leaks after a one stage operation died. The sole survivor underwent immediate proximal diverting colostomy plus drainage as the leak was quickly recognized.' All these anastomoses leaked between four and 16 days after a post-operative course that had been initially benign. They recommended that any leakage should be treated by colostomy and drainage, caecostomy being unreliable. A two- or three-stage procedure does this from the start.

Admittedly, staged procedures involve months of morbidity, three operations and great expense (about ten thousand dollars according to Rodkey and Welch, 1969), but their mortality is less. Furthermore, the very old and frail, who cannot withstand major surgery (Bolt, 1960), can be saved by the first stage. Later, if their condition improves after a colostomy, the feasibility of resection can be reviewed. One-stage resection puts the lives of a small proportion of patients at risk and should only be employed in carefully selected cases by those who specialize in colonic surgery.

(a) Elective Resection for Diverticulitis

Resection of the diseased bowel must follow drainage of an abscess and the establishment of a colostomy. The reasons for this have to be discussed.

A more difficult question is whether the colon should be removed after the resolution of an attack of diverticulitis which may or may not have been accompanied by a paracolic abscess that drained with conservative treatment. This decision may be difficult as surgeons are not prophets and the prognosis of diverticulitis is not known with certainty and one attack of diverticulitis is not followed, necessarily, by others (Bolt and Hughes, 1966; Bolt, 1973).

Physicians tend to the view that the disease has a good prognosis when treated medically and some have been critical of the fad of early resection of the sigmoid (Berman, Burdick, Heitzman and Prior, 1968). On the other hand, surgeons who have to cope with its dangerous complications believe that many cases of fistula and fatal peritonitis could have been avoided if patients with a long history of recurrent diverticulitis had been referred for a surgical opinion earlier. Undoubtedly, prophylactic resection of the sigmoid has saved lives and prevented much morbidity (Botsford and Zollinger, 1969; Colcock, 1971). A plea for planned surgery was made by Bacon and Magsanoc (1964) who reviewed 326 operations for diverticulitis performed between 1940 and 1963. They believed that diverticulitis led to surgery in at least 20% of patients and, by 1963, were operating on 70% of those referred to them. They had performed 45 staged resections involving 116 procedures with no deaths and 137 primary resections with two deaths, a mortality of 1·4%. They argued that this small mortality was acceptable when judged against the prolonged hospitalization involved in staged procedures. As a mortality of 8·1% resulted from emergency operations for complications, they advocated prophylactic elective resection in one or more stages. Bolt and Hughes (1966) and Parks and Connell (1970) found that about 30% of patients continued to have symptoms after an attack of diverticulitis whether they had been medically or surgically treated, but it was among the medically treated that severe bouts of recurrent pain occurred. Botsford and Zollinger (1969) pointed out that even those who only had mild symptoms never really felt well and that they were improved by resection. Colcock (1971) states that second attacks of diverticulitis are often worse than the first. Those who have recurrent symptoms which culminate in an emergency admission have a worse prognosis than do those whose first attack is unheralded by previous pain (Bolt and Hughes, 1966; Parks and Connell, 1970). Younger patients below the age of 50 with progressive disease have a particularly poor prognosis while those whose attack is preceded and followed by few symptoms are unlikely to develop complications (McGregor, Abernethy and Thomson, 1970; Bolt, 1973).

In the present state of our knowledge, the following factors have a bearing on whether to perform an elective resection or not.

(1) If a neoplasm cannot be excluded, operate as soon as is possible with safety.

(2) If an abscess has been drained or a colostomy fashioned, resection is indicated when the infection has settled.

(3) If the colonic lumen has been narrowed by diverticulitis or a barium enema outlines a track or an abscess cavity, the colon has been permanently damaged and is best resected.

(4) The prognosis is bad in patients with a long history of recurrent symptoms unless the colon is resected.

(5) Patients below 50 with recurrent symptoms are at risk and their lives may be altered for the better by timely surgery.

People in this group who often travel to places where medical facilities are few should be treated by elective resection.

(6) Obese patients are at a greater risk when complications develop. They should reduce weight so that elective resection can be performed safely. This chance should be taken; they tend to regain weight once they escape from medical supervision.

(7) Diabetics are particularly prone to complications.

(8) Persistent blood in the stools is an indication for surgery.

(9) Resection is contra-indicated if symptoms are due to painful diverticular disease. This will respond to a high fibre diet.

(10) Resection should be withheld in patients with one attack and no history of severe symptoms. They should be given a high fibre diet. The decision can be altered if symptoms persist or return.

(11) The old and frail should be treated by a high-fibre diet whenever possible as the disease tends to burn itself out in many of them. Furthermore many old people will not withstand major surgery.

In conclusion, diverticulitis and abscess formation are surgical emergencies that should be treated in hospital. Half these emergencies are preceded by less than a month's history (Hartley, 1964; Parks, 1969). A colon once damaged by inflammation, like an appendix, will probably give further trouble unless it is removed; this is especially true in the young. However, one attack of uncomplicated diverticulitis is not an indication for resection if only mild symptoms follow. The effect of a high-fibre diet should be tried after every attack of diverticulitis as this will cure symptoms in over 85% of patients providing no organic stenosis is present. The prognosis of the disease may be improved by the widespread adoption of this diet so that, except for the complications of diverticulitis, the need for surgery will be reduced (Painter, Almeida and Colebourne, 1972).

Chapter 15

Complicated Diverticular Disease: General Peritonitis

Acute diverticulitis may lead to perforation and to the formation of a small abscess but, if the perforation is large or the patient's defences are poor, peritonitis may spread rapidly. Perforation of diverticula in the caecum and transverse colon occurs on occasions, but in over 95% of cases, this dreaded complication originates in the thickened part of the sigmoid colon. Peritonitis due to diverticulitis often develops without warning, unheralded by previous symptoms. Acute diverticulitis gives rise to peritonitis in 1% to 17% of cases (Watkins and Oliver, 1966) and arose in 16·3% of 72 patients with diverticulitis in a Welsh general hospital (Staunton, 1962). In the United States, Smithwick (1960) reported that 13·4% of 545 patients with diverticulitis developed peritonitis. The hospital incidence of peritonitis due to diverticulitis was 14 cases compared with 1,402 patients with acute appendicitis, a ratio of 100 to 1 (Staunton, 1962); this corresponds with the figures of MacLaren (1957) namely that 26 patients with peritonitis due to diverticulitis were seen while 2,322 underwent emergency appendicectomy.

Obviously, no one surgeon will amass much personal experience of this emergency and this may account for 'the paucity of authoritative comment in the literature on this complication of diverticulitis' (MacLaren, 1957).

Diverticulitis may lead to spreading peritonitis which may be *purulent* or *faecal* in type, the latter being much the more lethal.

PURULENT PERITONITIS

This follows the infection of one or more diverticula, with or without abscess formation. Its presentation has been likened to 'left-sided appendicitis' but in old people, or when peritonitis spreads rapidly, all that can be diagnosed is the presence of peritonitis. It may mimic appendicitis whether or not the sigmoid crosses the midline and the correct pre-operative diagnosis was made only 33 times in 93 cases seen in a London hospital (Lyon, 1948; Dawson, Hanon and Roxburgh, 1965). This is because patients with generalized peritonitis frequently arrive in hospital so late that its cause cannot be diagnosed with certainty. Nevertheless, peritonitis due to diverticulitis should figure in the diagnosis in all patients who are over the age of 40, especially if they are known to have diverticulosis. The correct diagnosis is easier to make in the early stages when tenderness is limited to the left iliac fossa or if the pain started on the left or if guarding is maximal over the pelvic colon. A history of a recent enema or the taking of purgatives may be forthcoming (Ryan, 1964).

The temperature is usually raised but may be subnormal in patients who are old or shocked. Respiration may be embarrassed so that bronchitic patients become cyanosed. Fortunately their condition often improves under anaesthesia, which relieves pain and ventilates the lungs. Erect radiographs may show gas under the diaphragm but no ill patients should be x-rayed once it is certain that laparotomy is necessary. The rupture of a hitherto localized abscess may cause sudden spreading peritonitis and the rapid deterioration of the patient. Frequently the peritonitis seals off the perforation and it cannot be found at operation.

FAECAL PERITONITIS

Rupture of a diverticulum and the adjacent colonic wall produces a large perforation, through which bowel contents escape to produce faecal peritonitis. This catastrophe may occur following purgation, enemata or an attack of diarrhoea, or may be unheralded by any symptoms. The onset of pain is catastrophic and the patient often cannot be sure where the pain started. Board-like rigidity occurs early and shock is more marked than in purulent peritonitis; patients with faecal peritonitis often look extremely toxic and appear to be at death's door. The circulatory collapse is usually more profound than that seen in purulent peritonitis. Even the sudden rupture of a large abscess seldom causes the toxicity that follows faecal peritonitis.

Often the only diagnosis that can be made is peritonitis due to a ruptured viscus calling for urgent laparotomy, but the differential diagnosis should include other causes of peritonitis and infarction of the intestine.

PROGNOSIS OF PERITONITIS DUE TO DIVERTICULITIS

The mortality from peritonitis due to diverticulitis increases with age, as would be expected. Shocked patients have less chance of survival and a proportion of patients are so moribund that they are too ill to withstand the simplest surgery. Thus there is an irreducible mortality associated with this form of peritonitis, which may be as high as 15% (Dawson *et al.*, 1965).

The profound shock of faecal peritonitis may resemble that of gas gangrene, but the hope that this might respond to clostridial antitoxins has not been realized. The death rate from perforated peritonitis has dropped since 1935 owing to the introduction of sulphonamides, antibiotics, better anaesthesia and supportive therapy, but this fall in mortality from 72% to 13·6% applies only to purulent peritonitis. Faecal peritonitis remains just as lethal and still kills over half those who are struck down by it (MacLaren, 1957).

These figures are from MacLaren's excellent study of patients operated on between 1935 and 1955 at Edinburgh, when simple drainage, with or without colostomy, was the standard procedure. In recent years a more adventurous approach to this emergency has attempted to reduce the mortality. Most series are too small to prove the efficacy of the various procedures that have been advocated and so composite tables have been completed in the hope of showing how this dreaded complication should be tackled.

TREATMENT: GENERAL PRINCIPLES

The objects of treatment are fourfold:

(1) To resuscitate shocked patients for operation.
(2) To establish the diagnosis by laparotomy and to cleanse the peritoneal cavity thoroughly.
(3) To prevent further soiling of the peritoneum. This must guarantee that the perforation is closed and will remain

closed, which, in my experience, is impossible; or that it is removed from the abdominal cavity.

(4) To drain the abdomen and any abscess that is present.

Resuscitation begins with the emptying of the stomach by a naso-gastric tube. This makes the induction of anaesthesia safer and relieves the intense shock that attends acute dilatation of the stomach, that most dangerous feature of ileus due to peritonitis. Intravenous supportive therapy should begin at once and antibiotics are given intravenously so that an adequate dosage rapidly reaches the tissues.

Pain must be relieved as soon as peritonitis has been diagnosed; pethidine is the drug of choice. Peritonitis inhibits respiration and so the relief of pain often improves the pulse, blood pressure and respiration. Oxygen, digoxin, cortisone and vasopressors should be given to those whose condition still precludes the possibility of laparotomy.

Any beneficial effect that these measures produce usually becomes apparent fairly soon and it should be remembered that even cyanosed, shocked patients may rally still further under anaesthesia. This is because their pain is relieved and their lungs are ventilated with an adequate amount of oxygen.

Consequently, in borderline cases, the surgeon should err on the side of 'having a go'. The patient will lose his life if he fails to act.

Conservative treatment, namely the giving of antibiotics, analgesics, steroids, vasopressors, gastric suction and intravenous fluids should only be reserved for resuscitation. Conservative treatment by itself has no place in the treating of spreading peritonitis.

TREATMENT: OPERATIVE PROCEDURES

Sufficient access is gained through a paramedian incision. This will be on the left side if the correct diagnosis has been made. The sigmoid may appear to be almost normal with an obvious rent in it, but usually it is swollen and inflamed. Pus, faeces and even undigested fragments of food, such as tomato skins, may be found. The extent of the peritonitis is usually greater than in acute appendicitis. The appendix is often injected; this inflammation is secondary and is limited to its serosal surface. If a diagnosis of acute appendicitis has been followed by an incision over McBurney's point, the faecal odour of necrotic tissue will suggest the correct diagnosis quickly.

Good access is essential so a McBurney incision should be closed and a left paramedian incision should be made (Ryan, 1964; Staunton, 1962); this is unnecessary if the emergency procedure is to be limited to drainage. The establishment of a transverse colostomy requires a separate incision.

In purulent peritonitis, or in peritonitis due to the rupture of a pericolic abscess, often the perforation cannot be found as it has been sealed off by inflammation but, in faecal peritonitis, the perforation is larger and can usually be seen. The sigmoid and other viscera tend to be less inflamed in faecal than in purulent peritonitis.

After assessing the situation and endeavouring, sometimes with little success, to ascertain whether a carcinoma co-exists with diverticular disease, the surgeon has the choice of the following procedures:

(1) Drainage of the abdomen and peritoneal toilet.
(2) Drainage of the abdomen, peritoneal toilet and the establishment of a proximal colostomy.
(3) Exteriorization of the sigmoid colon together with the perforation; the exteriorized bowel is then opened to form a colostomy. This is combined with peritoneal toilet and drainage of the abdomen.
(4) Immediate resection of the sigmoid colon that bears the perforation. This may be achieved in one of three ways:—

(*a*) Resection of the perforation and adjacent colon by the Paul–Mikulicz technique;
(*b*) Resection of all the thickened inflamed sigmoid followed by bringing the open end of the proximal colon to the surface, to form a terminal colostomy, coupled with the closure of the lower bowel as in Hartman's procedure. This is accompanied by peritoneal toilet and drainage of the abdomen.
(*c*) Resection of the diseased bowel and its perforation followed by an immediate end-to-end anastomosis, together with peritoneal toilet and drainage of the abdomen.

The choice of procedure is still a vexed question. The results of surgery will be affected by the extent of the peritonitis found at operation. If laparotomy is performed for localized peri-colitis which would have resolved without surgery, then the procedure used will appear to carry a low mortality. As the indications for laparotomy vary from surgeon to surgeon this makes statistically significant information hard to come by (Killingback, 1970). The survival rate is also influenced by the surgeon's ability to operate both accurately and expeditiously.

In the past procedures (1) and (2) were accepted as adequate in the belief that sick patients could withstand only the mini-mum of surgery. At first, these procedures seemed successful as the mortality from peritonitis fell after the war. However, as many shocked patients with faecal peritonitis still succumb, more radical methods of dealing with this dire emergency have been tried in recent years.

PROCEDURE 1: DRAINAGE OF ABDOMEN AND PERITONEAL TOILET

Peritoneal toilet including lavage is essential, regardless of which surgical procedure is chosen. The peritoneum can dilute fluids such as pus, bile and gastric juice. This defence mechanism can be aided by washing out the abdomen with copious amounts of warm saline and by the instillation of 300 ml. of penicillin containing 50,000 units per ml. (Madden, 1966). Solid material such as faecoliths or fragments of food that escape from the colon act as foreign bodies and so it is essential to remove all particulate matter from the abdomen.

Faecal peritonitis is associated frequently with severe shock which may be caused by some unidentified and very toxic fraction of the faeces. Browne (1967) gave 2·5 g. of noxythiolin in 100 ml. of distilled water intraperitoneally to 11 patients with faecal peritonitis and only two died. Seven had perforated diverticulitis of whom one died on the tenth day from respiratory distress. Noxythiolin (noxyflex) slowly liberates formaldehyde and work on guinea-pigs suggests that it is of benefit (Browne and Stoller, 1970). The author has not used this drug but regards their treatment of 23 patients with faecal peritonitis with only three deaths as very encouraging. Pickard (1972) used larger doses of noxythiolin to wash out the peritoneum and to irrigate it post-operatively in two patients with diverticulitis; one old lady died of unrelated causes and the other recovered.

Repair of the perforation, in the hope that its closure will prevent further soiling of the peritoneum, seems logical but, in practice, suturing of the inflamed and oedomatous colon is unreliable (Staunton, 1962); in his series two of four patients treated by suture and drainage died. The late Sir Edward Muir considered that suturing the edges of a perforation was dangerous and used to wrap the perforation with omentum (Muir, 1966); omental patching is recommended by Tagart (1969) if only one diverticulum has perforated and the inflammation is very localized. The author believes that further faecal soiling can only be prevented by exteriorizing or by resecting the perforation and regards attempts to close it as a waste of time.

Drainage of the peritoneum allows pus and faecal matter to escape. The colon may perforate for a second time after surgery (Hayden, 1940); a corrugated drain alongside the sigmoid will lessen the effect of this complication. Drainage at one or more sites is an essential part of any operation for diverticulitis with peritonitis. Drainage alone is so simple that it enables surgeons of limited experience to operate rapidly. While it may be an adequate procedure when dealing with some cases of purulent peritonitis, it is a completely inadequate method of coping with faecal peritonitis or a patent perforation.

Recently, Bolt (1973) proposed that drainage without colostomy should become the standard operation for purulent peritonitis. He believes that the addition of a colostomy achieves nothing if the perforation is sealed and that it does not guarantee that pericolic inflammation will not continue unabated. Furthermore, he argues that, because the closure of a colostomy without prior resection is followed so often by a recurrence of symptoms, making a diversionary colostomy prejudices the need for resection and makes sigmoid colectomy almost inevitable.

It is difficult to argue with him as he has reported that about two thirds of 48 patients with purulent peritonitis were treated by drainage alone with a mortality of only 8 % (Bolt and Hughes, 1966), but it is my belief that a proximal colostomy should always be fashioned if the affected colon is not exteriorized or resected. I agree that simple drainage may sometimes be lifesaving in very sick patients, but wonder whether some patients who survive after simple drainage might have recovered if treated conservatively. A survey of the literature suggests that laparotomy is sometimes performed when the inflammatory process is still confined to the sigmoid's serosal surface and not from general peritonitis and so it may well be effective in the hands of those who operate early. Certainly there is no evidence that drainage alone is more or even equally as effective as drainage coupled with colostomy.

Furthermore, in my opinion, drainage alone is an inadequate method of dealing with a sigmoid that is oedematous and thickened or when it has formed the wall of a large abscess. Free perforation without faecal soiling has a mortality of 33·3% which is double that of purulent peritonitis with a closed perforation (MacLaren, 1957), and this may be because the infected sigmoid produces toxins which drain into the patient's circulation (Muir, 1966; Painter, 1970). In these cases, more aggressive surgery is needed and the grossly infected sigmoid should be resected just as one would remove a gangrenous appendix or gall-bladder. While drainage may be successful in mild purulent peritonitis, more radical surgery will be required if the present 10–15% mortality of this complication is to be further reduced (Botsford, Zollinger and Hicks, 1971).

Patients who recover from peritonitis after drainage must be investigated fully. Not all of them will require resection or myotomy as about half will experience only mild symptoms on their former diet. Patients under the age of 50 who have suffered from recurrent attacks of pain have a bad prognosis and these are candidates for resection but it is possible that their symptoms may be relieved by a high fibre diet including millers' bran. The effect of this diet on patients who have suffered from acute diverticulitis has yet to be evaluated but preliminary results are encouraging and suggest that only those with stenosis will need surgery (Painter, Almeida and Colebourne, 1972).

Finally, it must be emphasized that drainage by itself should never be used to treat faecal peritonitis or an open perforation. Most surgeons believe that it should be accompanied by a colostomy even when dealing with purulent peritonitis. The author has never relied on drainage alone and believes that the addition of a colostomy increases the survival rate and adds no significant risk to the emergency operation.

PROCEDURE 2: DRAINAGE TOGETHER WITH THE MAKING OF A TRANSVERSE COLOSTOMY

This is the most widely used method of treating peritonitis. Over the years, it has lessened the mortality of purulent
peritonitis to about 12% but this improvement is as much due
to the antibiotics and better supportive therapy as it is to the colostomy (MacLaren, 1957). Transverse colostomy should not be
used for faecal peritonitis as it leaves a column of faeces proximal
to an open perforation and these may escape and cause further
soiling; free perforations must be treated by a procedure that
excludes them from the peritoneum (Staunton, 1962; Smiley,
1966). Hence, the following discussion of the merits and
disadvantages of colostomy apply only to the treatment of
purulent peritonitis.

A diversionary colostomy should be made in the right half
of the transverse colon which is mobile and can be brought to
the surface easily. The left colon and splenic flexure is then left
free of adhesions to facilitate subsequent sigmoid colectomy.
Caecostomy is unreliable and should not be used. Some surgeons
have placed the colostomy near the perforation but if the sigmoid can be mobilized to an extent sufficient to allow this, then
it could be exteriorized or resected at the emergency operation.

A colostomy defunctions the distal bowel and allows it to rest
so that the inflammatory process resolves. The distal bowel can
then be resected with greater safety at a later date (Smithwick,
1942; Muir, 1966). Recently, Bolt (1973) has questioned this on
the grounds that a colostomy achieves nothing if the perforation
is sealed and once fashioned makes the future resection of the
colon almost inevitable. However, most surgeons of my
acquaintance are convinced that the distal colon recovers better
if it is defunctioned. Tagart (1969 and personal communication)
considers that a colostomy is often life-saving in purulent
peritonitis and the fact that faeces remain between it and the
inflamed sigmoid is of theoretical rather than practical importance. No controlled trial of the efficacy of drainage compared
with drainage and colostomy has been made and it is unlikely
that this will prove practicable in view of the variable presentation of the disease.

I believe that sound theoretical grounds exist for making a
colostomy. Cineradiographic studies show that the movement

of faeces from the proximal colon stimulate the sigmoid to segment and to generate pressure. Both these effects would hinder resolution and favour the rupture of a sealed perforation or of another diverticulum. Consequently, diversion of the faecal stream is as sound in principle as it is easy to perform. Furthermore, a colostomy relieves any unrecognized element of obstruction that may be present in the sigmoid and which may have contributed to the perforation and also decompresses the proximal intestine. This lessens the likelihood of distended bowel embarrassing the patient's respiration.

It is an accepted principle of war surgery that a colostomy should be made proximal to any injury of the large bowel so as to lessen the chances of subsequent necrosis and perforation. I believe that the same argument applies to the inflamed sigmoid whose wall is already weakened by a perforated diverticulum sealed only by fibrin. Even Bolt (1973) warns against handling the oedematous sigmoid in case this causes a faecal leak. Admittedly, a colostomy does not guarantee that a second perforation will not occur post-operatively and lead to fatal results (Hayden, 1940; Dawson *et al.*, 1965; Painter, 1970), but it cannot be claimed that the colostomy caused this disaster or that it would have been avoided by limiting the emergency operation to drainage alone. At present, experience teaches that a proximal colostomy should always be fashioned when draining purulent peritonitis unless more radical procedures are employed.

The second criticism of colostomy is that it prejudges the need for later resection because closure of colostomy without prior resection is followed frequently by a recurrence of symptoms. Bolt (1973) correctly maintains that this leads to some partial colectomies being performed that could be avoided. This criticism can be answered on two counts. The aim of the surgeon at the emergency operation is to save the life of a desperately ill patient and so the possible difficulties of later operations should not cloud his judgement or influence his choice of procedure. None of these problems will arise if the patient dies.

Second, although Smithwick (1942) pointed out that closure of a colostomy without prior resection gives poor results, this may not be so if cases are selected with care. I am indebted to Mr Louis de Jode for details of his experience. In the last seven years, he has performed 11 resections following colostomy for perforated diverticulitis and in the same period he has closed eight colostomies without resection having made sure that no organic stenosis of the sigmoid was present. The age of his patients ranges from 21 to 73 years (average 58) and the length of follow-up ranges from one to seven years (average 3·8). The colostomies were closed on average four months after the emergency operation for peritonitis. All seven patients are well and only one complains of mild symptoms. In two cases, resection was not performed because of the condition of the patients concerned, both of whom had other degenerative diseases. In the younger patients, de Jode could not bring himself to resect an almost normal colon with a lumen of normal diameter.

None of his patients were put on a low-residue diet and for the last three years he has prescribed a high fibre diet. Although it is too early to assess the long-term results of closure of colostomy without resection, his results suggest that this may be safe in selected cases if coupled with a high fibre diet. If this is so, the need for a three-stage resection will be reduced and lead to a great saving in hospital beds and money. Perforation followed by staged resection costs about $10,000 in the U.S.A., a price that few patients can afford (Rodkey and Welch, 1969). Hence, closure of colostomy without resection accompanied by a high-fibre diet deserves urgent assessment as it may lessen the morbidity attendant upon perforated diverticulitis.

The mortality of peritonitis due to diverticulitis, treated by drainage, with or without colostomy, is given in Table 14. Most authors do not define the type of peritonitis. On average, about one third succumb to this complication, although the mortality of purulent peritonitis has dropped to around 10%, while faecal peritonitis still kills two thirds of its victims. The author has treated over 30 patients by drainage and colostomy with an overall mortality of 33%. All of his cases of faecal peritonitis died and 16% of these with purulent peritonitis. These results leave much to be desired and have prompted colonic surgeons to attack the problem with the more radical means described below.

PROCEDURE 3: EXTERIORIZATION OF THE SIGMOID COLON AND THE PERFORATION

Drainage with or without colostomy may be followed by further leakage and this has been avoided by exteriorization of

TABLE 14

MORTALITY OF PERITONITIS CAUSED BY DIVERTICULITIS
WHEN TREATED BY LAPAROTOMY AND DRAINAGE
WITH OR WITHOUT A PROXIMAL COLOSTOMY

Author and Date	Number of Cases	Deaths	Mortality %
MacLaren (1957)	65	27	41·4
Ryan (1958)	5	2	40·0
Brown and Toomey (1960)	41	20	50·0
Smiley (1960)	16	9	56·2
Dawson, Hanon & Roxburgh (1965)	61	19	31
Bolt and Hughes (1966)	52	7	13·0
Beard and Gazet (1961)	18	3	16·6
Staunton (1962)	9	4	44·4
Hartley (1964)	15	5	33·3
Madden (1966)	20	7	35·0
Muir (1966)	35	5	14·3
Tagart (1969)	7	2	28·6
Botsford, Zollinger and Hicks (1971)	11	11	100·0
Byrne and Garick (1971)	13	2	15·0
Miller & Wichern (1971)	14	2	14·0
Totals:	382	124	37·7%

(1) Madden (1966) collected a series of 267 patients treated in this manner with 126 deaths, a mortality of 47·1%.

(2) MacLaren (1957) found that even in the antibiotic era the mortality from faecal peritonitis remained at over 60% but had dropped to 13·6% for purulent peritonitis.

(3) Bolt and Hughes (1966) recorded a 75% mortality in 4 patients with faecal peritonitis but only 8% in 48 with purulent peritonitis.

(4) The other authors do not make clear which type of peritonitis was present. This may account for the variation in their results.

the perforation after lavage and drainage (Table 15). Mobilization of the sigmoid can be difficult when the mesocolon is contracted by fibrosis, but is possible in almost every case with patience, if the peritoneum lateral to colon is incised along the 'white line' and the operation does not hesitate to mobilize the rectum (Staunton, 1962). Dissection with the finger is safe when the tissues are oedematous and ligation of the sigmoid vessels allows the sigmoid to be brought to the surface and held in position by one or two glass rods. The wound is closed around it in layers and dressed with vaseline gauze. The perforation will heal in a few days (Linder and Hoffman, 1962) but I prefer to open it widely so that any obstruction is relieved before the patient leaves the operating theatre. This procedure lowers the intracolonic pressure and ensures that no further peritoneal soiling will occur. In about three weeks, the appendices epiploica have disappeared and the healthy granulating colon can be resected. It is important to remove all the thickened colon and recto-sigmoid junction and not merely the loop that is outside the abdomen. The intraperitoneal anastomosis is accompanied by a drain and, unless a proximal colostomy is deemed necessary, the patient is cured in two operations. This method of dealing with the emergency can be used for both purulent and faecal peritonitis and is followed by a very smooth convalescence as compared with the morbidity of three stage procedures. Staunton (1962) echoed this view and advised immediate resection in the few cases where exteriorization proved to be impossible.

Exteriorization removes the perforation from the peritoneum but leaves the suppurating sigmoid to pour its toxic products into the patient's circulation. Obviously, this can only be prevented by immediate resection, but Dendy Moore (1964) has described a 'half-way' procedure in which the exteriorized part of the sigmoid is resected after the abdomen has been closed. This technique removes both the perforation and most of the septic sigmoid; in the words of Moore, 'the more serious the condition of the patient, the more necessary is it to prevent resoiling.'

The results of exteriorization are given in Table 15.

TABLE 15

MORTALITY OF PERITONITIS CAUSED BY DIVERTICULITIS
WHEN TREATED BY EXTERIORIZATION OF THE SIGMOID COLON
AND THE PERFORATION

Author and Date	Number of Cases	Deaths	Mortality %
MacLaren (1957)	7	3	42·9
Staunton (1962)	5	0	0
Smiley (1966)	3	0	0
Watkins and Oliver (1966)	7	0	0
Roxburgh, Dawson and Yeo (1968)	1	1	100
Tagart (1969)	2	0	0
Rodkey and Welch (1969)	2	0	0
Totals:	27	4	14·8%

PROCEDURE 4: EMERGENCY RESECTION
OF THE SIGMOID COLON

The mortality of diverticulitis with peritonitis is so high when treated by simple measures that it has been realized that it is the disease and not the emergency surgery that kills the patient. Hence, there has been a change to more radical surgery, not only in faecal but also in purulent peritonitis with a patent perforation. Ryan (1964) emphasized that cellulitis of the sigmoid, which has been called 'gangrenous sigmoiditis' must be resected as soon as possible but not necessarily with immediate anastomosis. Several surgeons have been impressed by the clinical improvement in their patients that follows resection of the toxic bowel (Belding, 1957; Madden and Tan, 1961; Large, 1964; Ryan, 1965; Madden, 1966; Roxburgh *et al.*, 1968; Dandekar and McCann, 1969; Moore, 1969; Byrne and Garick, 1971). Resection not only relieves obstruction and prevents further leakage but also removes the septic focus of infection. The open ends of the colon are exteriorized as a terminal colostomy and a mucous fistula or brought together by the Paul-Mickulicz technique. Alternatively, the distal end can be closed as in Hartman's procedure. Continuity of the colon is restored later at a second operation, but this can be avoided if emergency resection is followed immediately by intraperitoneal anastomosis, so that the emergency and definitive treatment of the disease is combined in one operation. Unfortunately, this ideal procedure carries risks which cannot be ignored.

The Paul-Mickulicz technique resects the perforation and adjacent bowel. It may involve extensive mobilization of the sigmoid, but the retroperitoneal tissue planes can be opened without complications (Roxburgh *et al.*, 1968). In my opinion, exteriorization is equally possible once the sigmoid is mobilized and is simpler, quicker and more effective, especially if the colon outside the abdomen is resected by Moore's method. Both operations fail to remove all the thickened sigmoid and must be followed by myotomy or resection. If this thickening is limited to the immediate vicinity of the perforation the Paul-Mickulicz resection is useful (Tagart, 1969) but such cases are not common. The results of these procedures are given in Table 16.

EMERGENCY RESECTION WITH IMMEDIATE ANASTOMOSIS

This ideal procedure saves time and expense but it cannot be attained with an acceptable mortality except by a few experienced colonic surgeons. Belding (1957) and Ryan (1958) reported its successful use but it was brought into prominence by the arguments of Madden and Tan (1961) who treated perforations, whether from cancer or diverticulitis, by this method. They collected figures showing that an immediate resection had a lower mortality than drainage and colostomy and were convinced that 'the rapidity of clinical improvement and the lessened morbidity after primary resection compared with patients after a first-stage procedure have been most impressive'. They attributed this to the removal of the source of the contamination.

Resection is easier if it is sufficiently extensive to allow the anastomosis to be made through relatively normal colon. Tension must be avoided by mobilization of the proximal colon (Rodkey and Welch, 1969). Every anastomosis should be drained; the track thus formed allows any leakage from the anastomosis to escape. If the rectum is mobilized, such faecal fistula occur more often and then the suture line should be protected by a colostomy. The outer layer of sutures should be unabsorbable (Madden and Tan, 1961; Madden, 1966) and Large (1964) went so far as to use a single layer of stainless steel sutures.

Madden's contention that immediate resection lowers the mortality from peritonitis has been supported by the experience of others both here and in the United States of America (Table 16). This radical approach can reduce the mortality to less than 10% and this is impressive considering that this procedure tends to be used more in faecal peritonitis.

IMMEDIATE ANASTOMOSIS

Emergency resection has been justified by the results obtained by expert colonic surgeons but this fact should not be used as an excuse for the wholesale practice of immediate anastomosis by the rest of us. Even worse would be the adoption of this practice by young surgeons still in training as this would result

TABLE 16

MORTALITY OF PERITONITIS CAUSED BY DIVERTICULITIS
WHEN TREATED BY EMERGENCY RESECTION AND
IMMEDIATE ANASTOMOSIS, WITH OR WITHOUT
PROXIMAL COLOSTOMY

Author and Date	Number of Cases	Deaths	Mortality %
Belding (1957)	3	0	0
Large (1964)	18	2	11·1
Ryan (1965)	7	0	0
Madden (1966)	25	2	8·0
Roxburgh, Dawson and Yeo (1968)	8	1	12·5
Dandekar and McCann (1969)	7	1	14·3
Rodkey and Welch (1969)	8	0	0
Tagart (1969)	11	0	0
Whelan, Furcinitti and Lavarreda (1971)	5	1	20
Byrne and Garick (1972)	2	0	0
Totals:	94	7	7·46%

Note: (1) Madden (1966) collected a series of 85 patients so treated with 8 deaths, a mortality of 9·4%
(2) Both Large (1964) and Madden (1966) included cases which were found to have perforated due to carcinoma of the colon.

in a needlessly high mortality (Bolt, 1973). Not only is it difficult to suture the swollen sigmoid safely but faecal soiling and infection favour the disruption of anastomoses (Hawley, 1973) and while rapid resection may improve the condition of sick patients, they cannot withstand the added burden of the prolonged surgery attendant upon a technically difficult anastomosis.

Whelan and his colleagues (1971) agreed with Madden that the toxic sigmoid should be resected but fought shy of immediate anastomosis if peritonitis was well established or if the proximal colon was loaded with faeces, because both factors endangered the integrity of the suture line. The advantage of immediate anastomosis is lost if a colostomy is necessary at the time of operation or has to be fashioned because the suture line leaks. This may occur in planned resection between 5 and 16 days post-operatively with little warning and proved fatal in four out of five patients, the fifth being saved by a timely colostomy. By contrast, five leaking anastomoses after resection came to no harm as they had been protected by a colostomy (Botsford and Zollinger, 1969). The early detection of dehiscence of the suture line may be difficult at the best of times but is even more difficult when the clinical signs are confused not only by the emergency operation but also by peritonitis. Some have estimated that faecal fistula follows one stage anastomosis in 25% of cases and so a colostomy is often not only wise but also necessary.

Hence, even the expert would be wise to fashion a colostomy when performing immediate anastomosis. If this argument is accepted, then the patient is not cured by one operation and the great advantage of emergency anastomosis is lost.

EMERGENCY RESECTION WITH DELAYED ANASTOMOSIS

This is gaining favour because it removes the septic focus and does not involve the making of an anastomosis under less than ideal conditions. Moore (1969) described an 'exteriorization–resection' technique which was successful in 15 patients. This removes most of the inflamed bowel, relieves obstruction and exteriorizes the perforation. It is simple and should be within the capability of a young surgeon in training who faces this emergency in the middle of the night.

Alternatively, both open ends of the remaining colon can be brought to the surface. This may be impossible if the remaining lower bowel is too short when it must be closed as in Hartman's procedure. Ryan (1964) recommends that this closed stump should be attached to the anterior sacro-iliac ligaments with black silk sutures. These are cut long to facilitate its identification at a later laparotomy. Hartman's procedure is simpler and safer than anastomosis or even a Paul-Mickulicz resection. The subsequent restoration of the colon's continuity may be difficult due to adhesions (Tagart, 1969) but, in my opinion, this consideration should not influence the surgeon during the emergency operation, the object of which is to save life.

The results of resection without anastomosis are given in Table 17. The numbers are small and include Moore's series. Whelan and his colleagues (1971) favour this method because they reported that two out of six primary anastomoses gave way,

TABLE 17

MORTALITY OF PERITONITIS CAUSED BY DIVERTICULITIS
WHEN TREATED BY EMERGENCY RESECTION WITHOUT
IMMEDIATE ANASTOMOSIS: THIS INCLUDES RESECTION BY THE
PAUL-MICKULICZ METHOD

Author and Date	*Number of Cases*	*Deaths*	*Mortality %*
MacLaren (1957)	1	0	0
Roxburgh, Dawson and Yeo (1968)			
(1) Immediate Resection	8	1	12·5
(2) Paul-Mickulicz Resection	8	0	0
Moore (1969)	15	0	0
Ryan (1969)	1	0	0
Tagart (1969)	3	0	0
Whelan, Furcinitti and Laverreda (1971)	4	1	25%
Totals:	40	2	5%

Note: Moore employed exteriorization of the perforation and then excised the part of the colon which was outside the abdomen after closing the abdominal wall round it.

but both patients were saved by timely intervention in the form of Hartman's procedure. The author has used this method successfully in four cases and twice in coping with the disruption of a low anastomosis. As this complication is so similar to the situation that exists immediately after emergency resection of the sigmoid, he believes that the exteriorization of the cut ends of the colon or Hartman's procedure should be given a trial as it promises to be the method of choice in dealing with this emergency. This is the view of Miller and Wichern (1971) who treated four patients successfully in this manner. They restored the continuity of the colon after an interval of three and ten weeks; all four patients recovered smoothly. They admitted that a one-stage operation is the ideal, but sensibly concluded that immediate anastomosis is an additional risk in an already debilitated patient.

CONCLUSION

The results of the treatment of peritonitis due to diverticulitis are difficult to assess because the presentation of this complication is so variable. For example, a 40-year-old man was observed for four days while his left-sided pain almost disappeared. He suddenly became shocked due to the rupture of a pericolic abscess and died four hours after drainage and colostomy. By contrast, an 85-year-old man with severe generalized pain and a rigid silent abdomen was only slightly shocked. I exteriorized his sigmoid together with a perforation two inches long which had allowed four hard balls of faeces to escape into the peritoneum. The degree of peritonitis was minimal and his recovery was smooth. His sigmoid was resected four weeks later.

The memory of a 40-year-old dying of purulent peritonitis and an 80-year-old surviving faecal peritonitis prompts me to question whether the division of peritonitis into 'faecal' and 'purulent' may be too rigid. MacLaren (1957) did a great service in introducing this classification which drew attention to the poor prognosis of faecal peritonitis. However, the prognosis is also affected by the degree of shock and, whichever type of peritonitis is present, this is determined by the degree of sepsis, the organism concerned and *the mass of the tissue that is infected.*

It would appear that drainage may be all that is necessary if only pus is present but immediate resection is necessary if the sigmoid is nearly gangrenous. These more desperate emergencies demand more radical surgery if more patients are to survive while those with minimal sepsis will survive when treated by a simpler procedure.

Although no hard and fast rules can be laid down, an attempt will be made to define the indications for the procedures that have been described.

Simple drainage should be reserved for mild purulent peritonitis. It should never be used for faecal peritonitis or gross inflammation of the sigmoid.

Drainage and colostomy should be used for purulent peritonitis. It should not be used for faecal peritonitis or severe pericolitis. It is easy to perform and can be used by the occasional surgeon.

Exteriorization with or without Moore's type of resection, appears to give the best results for both beginners and experts. It removes the perforation from the abdomen but does not remove all the septic focus from the circulation.

Emergency resection with delayed anastomosis should be used by both expert and beginner for gross sigmoiditis or for a free perforation. Resection by the Mickulicz method is not so simple and should be reserved for a perforation occurring in diverticular disease that is limited to a few segments of the colon.

Emergency resection with immediate anastomosis yields excellent results when successfully performed. The risks involved are high and post-operative complications common, dangerous and difficult to detect. This procedure should only be used by experts in colonic surgery and even they would be wise to protect their anastomosis with a colostomy in about a quarter of their patients.

Chapter 16

Complicated Diverticular Disease: Fistula Formation

The sigmoid and its mesocolon may become adherent to neighbouring structures due to recurrent attacks of diverticulitis or following abscess formation. A paracolic abscess may burst into the bladder, ureter, renal pelvis, vagina or into the small bowel. An abscess may point to the skin surface and burst through the abdominal wall or perineum but, nowadays, colocutaneous fistula are almost always the result of surgical interference.

(1) VESICO-COLIC FISTULA

These fistula should really be called colo-vesical fistula as, in the main, the flow of contents is from the colon to the bladder. Jones (1859) first described this complication of diverticulitis at a time when such fistula were caused most commonly by cancer, tuberculosis or foreign bodies such as fishbones ulcerating through the colonic wall (Cripps, 1888). As diverticular disease became commoner, this complication was recognized by Beer (1904) and by Moynihan (1907) and today from 6% to 23% of patients operated on for diverticulitis suffer from vesico-colic fistula (Berman and Kirsner, 1972). At the Mayo Clinic, between 1939 and 1949, 202 patients were treated surgically for diverticulitis and 46 (22·8%) had this type of fistula (Mayo and Blunt, 1950). These figures are not representative as this clinic attracts difficult surgical problems. In a busy general hospital only ten out of 258 patients had fistula of any kind, and only three of these involved the bladder (Brown and Toomey, 1960) and Patterson (1951) reported an incidence of less than 2% in 434 patients. Obviously no general surgeon gains much experience of dealing with this condition; the author has dealt with five cases.

Vesico-colic fistula is three to five times more common in men than in women as the uterus tend to keep the bladder and colon apart, but the incidence in the sexes is equal when only women who have undergone hysterectomy are considered (Lockhart–Mummery, 1958).

Clinical picture. These fistula may be heralded by recurrent attacks of cystitis without pneumaturia and so patients are often referred to urologists, the condition being unsuspected. Alternatively, the first symptom may be an episode of intense cystitis which settles down and cystoscopy may reveal a granulomatous polypoid mass which resembles a carcinoma of the bladder. The classical presenting symptom of this complication is pneumaturia with or without the passing of faecal matter in the urine. This makes the diagnosis and the problem then remains of diagnosing the nature of the lesion. The passage of urine from the rectum is much less common.

An untreated fistula has a bad prognosis as, in most cases, recurrent attacks of cystitis lead to a contracted bladder, stone formation, ascending pyelitis and death. However, a few patients are remarkably tolerant of fistula and, apart from occasional attacks of cystitis, remain well for many years (Lockhart–Mummery, 1958; Ewell, 1961). This complication has been found in patients as young as 24 and may occur at any later age; on average it is seen in the early fifties (Mayo and Blunt, 1950).

The Diagnosis is usually made on the history of pneumaturia. Investigations include cystoscopy, which may reveal a fistula, but often a poor view is obtained because the bladder is injected and only granulation tissue but not the fistula is seen. Biopsy may prove that this tissue is neoplastic but a negative biopsy is inconclusive. Sigmoidoscopy must be performed but is usually unhelpful except to exclude the presence of a low carcinoma. The air insufflated into the bowel may later be passed per urethra and this will confirm the presence of a fistula but will not help to decide its nature. A cystogram may result in dye appearing in the bowel. A contrast enema performed with barium or gastrograffin seldom demonstrates the fistula but is essential to show the nature of the colonic disease. The urine should be centrifuged as this may show faecal debris and muscle fibres and it should be cultured for spores. An enema containing methylene blue may be followed by the passage of green urine thus demonstrating the presence of a fistula.

The Differential Diagnosis is between diverticular disease, carcinoma and Crohn's disease; other causes are very rare in this country. The diagnosis may be obvious but sometimes the differentiation is extremely difficult and may be impossible before operation. An intravenous pyelogram should be performed not only as a test of renal function but to exclude a nephro-colic or uretero-colic fistula. If the fistula is seen at cystoscopy, transurethral biopsy may reveal its nature. The larger the fistula the more likely it is to be malignant; but an inflammatory fistula may be surrounded by exuberant granulation tissue. A barium enema may reveal diverticulosis with a rigid segment that fails to relax with probanthine, but even this may be due to benign fibrosis converting an adherent colon into a rigid tube. Rectal and vesical washings may be helpful but often skilled pathologists find it difficult to give a dogmatic opinion as to the nature of such specimens. If there is any doubt as to whether the fistula is benign, operation must take place as soon as possible.

The treatment of this complication is surgical and consists of separating the bladder and colon. The bladder is then closed with an indwelling urethral catheter which remains in position for a week. The bladder heals without difficulty in almost every case.

The diseased colon must be resected; ideally this should be performed in one stage but the operation should be staged if the patient's condition is poor, if the amount of inflammatory tissue around the fistula makes resection difficult or if an abscess is present. Ewell (1961) cured his patients in one operation as did Mayo and Blunt (1950). However, the latter favoured the fashioning of a colostomy in difficult cases and stressed that if a colostomy is made prior to resection, it must be double-barrelled to allow the distal inflammation to subside.

Ideally, the sigmoid can be resected without a colostomy so that the patient is cured in one operation (Ewell, 1961). Unfortunately, inflammatory adhesions may be so extensive that it is technically difficult and hazardous to attempt a cure in one operation. It is then wise to perform a proximal colostomy and this should be a defunctioning colostomy (Mayo and Blunt, 1950). If the anastomosis is difficult or has to be made in the vicinity of an abscess cavity, it is wise to protect it with a colostomy which can be closed in about three weeks. Operations for vesico-colic fistula frequently necessitate a low anastomosis.

This may be difficult and discretion dictates that a colostomy should be made. The pelvis should be drained post-operatively and antibiotics given to suppress the urinary infection.

If the presence of a carcinoma is suspected, resection must be carried out at almost any cost and the bladder closed. If continuity of the colon cannot be restored immediately, the lower end should be closed as in Hartman's procedure and the upper end brought out as a terminal colostomy. The mesocolon, lymphatics, and blood vessels must be resected as in an operation for cancer.

Each case differs and the operation must be staged or modified to meet the complications encountered. Diverticular disease is a benign condition and the surgeon must play for safety at all times unless the presence of a carcinoma is suspected. Conservative treatment of a vesico-colic fistula is indicated in the old and frail. Modern chemotherapy will control recurrent urinary infection and allow them to finish their lives without the disadvantages of a permanent colostomy. This would be the fate of those who were unfit to withstand resection but, fortunately, few people come into this category today. A preliminary colostomy may improve debilitated patients by causing their urinary infection to subside so that resection can be undertaken.

The place of myotomy in the treatment of vesico-colic fistula was discussed briefly at the Royal Society of Medicine on 27th March 1974. Mr Michael Reilly had performed a sigmoid myotomy with closure of the perforation in place of resection but a fistula had resulted and he did not advise that this procedure should be used for this complication. Mr Peter Lord pointed out that the bladder defect was easy to close. The pressure differential ensured that material would flow from the colon to the bladder and for this reason such fistula should be termed 'colo-vesical' and not 'vesico-colic'. Hence, it was his opinion that an adequate myotomy extending below the recto-sigmoid junction would relieve any functional obstruction in the sigmoid and lead to the cure of the fistula between the colon and bladder.

It has been shown that myotomy lowers the intracolinic pressure and this manoeuvre has been used as an adjunct to uretero-colic anastomosis with good effect (Daniel and Singh, 1969) so that further experience may show that myotomy has a place in the treatment of vesico-colic fistula. In the author's opinion, this is of academic interest only because closure of the bladder and resection of the sigmoid are both well tried procedures that yield excellent results with an acceptable mortality. There is as yet no evidence that myotomy lowers either the mortality or the morbidity of vesico-colic fistula operations and so there is no justification for its use by general surgeons.

The treatment of uretero-colic fistula and fistula between the left colon and the renal pelvis rests on the same principles, namely, separation of the involved organs and resection of the diseased colon. The location of such fistula is difficult to find and may require repeated cineradiographic studies. The author treated a vesico-colic fistula only to find that a gastro-graffin enema outlined the left renal pelvis. Attempts to demonstrate the precise position of the connection between the left colon and ureter were undertaken at the Royal Marsden Hospital by Mr Cyril Cooling but its exact site could not be demonstrated by cineradiography. It was decided to observe the patient after his urine had been made sterile with antibiotics. He has remained well for five years and has not suffered an attack of cystitis during this time. It is presumed that this second fistula has closed and this happy result may have been partly due to the administration of a high fibre diet.

Sigmoid diverticulitis may cause an abscess which obstructs the left ureter and leads to hydronephrosis without establishing a connection between the colon and ureter (Hersch and Schwabe, 1963). This is another reason why pyelography should be performed in patients with diverticulitis.

(2) COLO-VAGINAL FISTULA

A colo-vaginal fistula results in the passage of air, faeces and pus per vaginam. Such a fistula may be caused not only by diverticulitis but also by carcinoma of the colon or cervix or following irradiation for cervical cancer. The investigation and treatment of this condition are similar to those outlined for a vesico-colic fistula. The treatment is surgical unless the tissues are so damaged by the infiltration of malignant cells or the effects of radiotherapy that they are unlikely to heal. It is wise to precede the definitive operation by establishing a colostomy and to perform a descending pyelogram, not only for the reasons already mentioned but also because obstruction of a ureter may lead to the detection of an unsuspected carcinoma.

Damage to a ureter that is involved in inflammatory tissue may be avoided by passing a ureteric catheter prior to laparotomy as this can be palpated at operation to define the precise course of the ureter.

(3) ENTERO-COLIC AND COLO-CUTANEOUS FISTULA

Both require similar investigations. The former may not be demonstrated without cineradiographic studies and colo-cutaneous fistula are nearly always the result of the surgical drainage of a pericolic abscess. Neither will heal until the diseased bowel has been resected and, if a colostomy has been made, this should not be closed until after resection or myotomy. The presence of a carcinoma or of Crohn's disease must be excluded in all such cases.

Chapter 17

Complicated Diverticular Disease: Obstruction

Symptoms of intestinal obstruction are present in about one quarter of patients with diverticulitis who require admission to hospital (Guy and Werelius, 1952; Brown and Toomey, 1969). This complication may be due to fibrosis of the sigmoid caused by recurrent attacks of diverticulitis or to ileus due to pus in the peritoneal cavity. Organic narrowing of the colon due to scarring may produce a stricture which cannot relax even after propantheline has been given (Lumsden and Truelove, 1959). This may make it difficult or impossible to be sure whether the resultant obstruction is due to diverticulitis or to cancer.

In 1904, Beer described six cases of stenosis caused in this way and Mayo, Wilson and Giffen (1907) reported five 'tumours' of the sigmoid due to diverticulitis that had been resected and claimed that this was the first time that diverticula had been demonstrated in living patients. Moynihan (1907a and b) removed six such 'tumours' in three years believing that he was dealing with cancer. He remarked that this ability of diverticulitis to mimic cancer probably accounted for some of the 'cures' of malignant disease that had been reported. It is worth remembering that, up to the Second World War, surgeons were unwilling to resect the colon for benign conditions because the operation carried at least a 10%, if not a 25% mortality (Rankin, 1930).

CLINICAL FEATURES

The presenting symptoms and the diagnosis of obstruction needs no description here. It may be caused by thickening of the colonic wall with infolding of the mucosa to which has been added fibrosis from recurrent attacks of diverticulitis and also by adhesions forming between the large and small bowel (Brown and Toomey, 1960). Fibrosis of the mesocolon leading to the kinking of the sigmoid may contribute to sub-acute obstruction (Patton, 1953). Subacute obstruction develops slowly so that the diagnosis can be made at leisure by sigmoidoscopy, barium studies and by colonoscopy if this is available. Sigmoidoscopy will exclude a growth in the lowest part of the large bowel but seldom yields a definite diagnosis. It should be performed with great care and no attempt to pass the instrument further should be made if it causes pain as this can be dangerous.

Obstruction due to ileus is much commoner than organic stenosis (Tagart, 1969). It is caused by local or general peritonitis involving the small bowel. It disappears when the underlying infection resolves. This can be aided by gastric suction, intravenous therapy and antibiotics or the drainage of an abscess. Bevan (1961) reported that 13 out of 16 patients with this complication were relieved by conservative treatment while the other three required surgery.

THE DIFFERENTIAL DIAGNOSIS OF OBSTRUCTION

It may be very difficult to determine the nature of an organic obstruction. It is often not certain whether cancer co-exists with diverticulitis even after the abdomen has been opened and the inflammatory mass inspected (Reilly, 1967; Colcock, 1971). Nevertheless, it is most important to endeavour to make the correct diagnosis before operation and this is usually possible as radiology is accurate in about 90% of cases in differentiating between the two conditions (Ponka, Fox and Brush, 1959). If the diagnosis of diverticulitis is certain, the surgeon can afford to wait and observe the effects of conservative treatment or to see whether an inflammatory mass resolves after a proximal colostomy has been made. On the other hand, if carcinoma of the colon cannot be excluded, resection must take place within a month at the latest. If the nature of the problem is still uncertain at laparotomy the surgeon must decide whether to undertake an extensive resection of the sigmoid together with its lymphatic glands or to perform a lesser procedure. When in doubt he must assume that the obstruction is malignant and proceed accordingly.

This problem is common and will become more frequent in an ageing population. Ponka, Fox and Brush (1959), calculated that 20 million Americans would be over the age of 65 in 1975 and that between 100,000 and 150,000 of them would require surgery for diverticulitis and that about 5% of these would be found to have cancer of the colon as well as diverticula. In their 355 cases of colonic cancer, 75 (21%) had diverticula as well and when the sigmoid region was considered no less than 56 of 197 patients with cancer had diverticula, an incidence of 28%. Both diseases are becoming commoner and so they will exist together in the same patient with increasing frequency (Fig. 60).

DISTRIBUTION THROUGOUT THE LARGE BOWEL

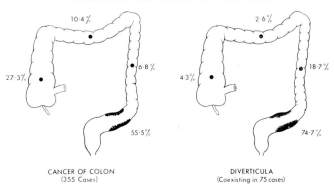

CANCER OF COLON
(355 Cases)

DIVERTICULA
(Coexisting in 75 cases)

FIG. 60. Diagram to show how cancer and diverticular disease frequently coexist as both are common diseases (after Ponka, Fox and Brush 1959).

The early diagnosis appears to have a bearing on prognosis. Mayo reported that the five-year survival rate of patients with colonic neoplasms and diverticula was only 39% compared with 52% when a carcinoma was present by itself (Berman and Kirsner, 1972). Whether this is due to operation being delayed because symptoms which would otherwise have led to the discovery of cancer were attributed to diverticulitis is not certain, but this is a possible explanation of these findings.

Clinically, there are some differences in the presentation of colonic cancer and diverticulitis but these are of academic interest only because it is impossible to be certain on clinical grounds alone that an obstruction is benign. Cramp-like pain in the left iliac fossa becomes progressively worse if caused by cancer; it is intermittent in diverticulitis and occurs in a greater proportion of patients. Two thirds of patients with cancer bleed compared with 30% in diverticulitis and the passage of mucus is much

commoner in malignant disease. Cancer should always be considered to be present until excluded if a palpable mass is present
or if a mass fails to diminish in size after colostomy. Carcinoma
tends to involve only one or two segments of the colon while
inflammatory scarring tends to involve a greater length of the
bowel. The duration of symptoms may be a few years in
diverticulitis but a history of only nine months is the average
for cancer. Perforation with abscess formation occurs in up to
one third of cases of diverticulitis but is seen in less than 10% of
those with malignant disease. As would be expected, fever is
commoner in diverticulitis (Welch and Rodkey, 1956; Rodkey
and Welch, 1959; Ponka, Fox and Brush, 1959, 1960; Colcock,
1972).

The differences are too small to enable a clinical diagnosis to
be made with confidence and radiology must be employed and
when possible together with exfoliative cytology. The radiological features of the two conditions have been described in
Chapter 4 but some doubt as to the true diagnosis will remain
in some 15% of patients even after barium studies have been
carried out. Consequently, it is essential that obstruction is
assumed to be malignant until it is proved otherwise. In particular, when patients who are known to have diverticular
disease complain of symptoms, these must never be attributed
to the disease until the presence of a carcinoma has been ruled
out. Any change in the frequency or the severity of any previous
symptoms must be investigated as a matter of urgency as this
may indicate that a neoplasm has developed in an area of
diverticulitis. This is not because cancer is 'grafted on to'
diverticulosis, to use Mayo's phrase, but because the two conditions have the same epidemiology and affect the same age
group. They might be said to grow in the same soil because both
afflict those Western nations whose diet is fibre-deficient and
who pass small viscous stools (Cleave, Campbell and Painter,
1969; Burkitt, Walker and Painter, 1972 and 1974).

THE SURGICAL TREATMENT OF OBSTRUCTION

This follows first principles; an organic stricture must be
resected. If obstruction develops slowly, it can be investigated
and a planned resection performed in one or more stages. The
decision as to whether to stage the operation will be made for

the reasons discussed elsewhere but, again, it should be stressed that a colostomy should be made if any difficulty is experienced in making the anastomosis, as if infection endangers its integrity.

Acute obstruction should be treated by colostomy and later resection. The safety of staged procedures is well proven; a colostomy allows the inflammation to resolve so that the empty sigmoid can be resected as a planned procedure. Furthermore, this conservative approach allows the extent of the disease to be assessed by barium enema after the emergency has passed. It is often surprising to find that less sigmoid is narrowed than appeared to be the case at the initial laparatomy when inflammation and oedema made the whole sigmoid colon rigid and thickened. The colostomy is closed after the distal bowel has been resected or its lumen widened by myotomy. If the presence of a carcinoma is suspected or proven by a later barium enema, resection must follow within one month of the emergency operation.

In recent years, there has been a tendency to resect at once if the obstruction is thought to be malignant. The continuity of the colon is restored at once or at a later date. An anastomosis even in acute obstruction has yielded excellent results in experienced hands but I believe that a proximal colostomy should be fashioned to protect any suture line made under these adverse circumstances. Reilly (1967) advises surgeons to attempt to mobilize an obstructive mass and has emphasized that this is usually possible even in apparently unpromising cases. Even when perforation has occurred near a carcinoma and an abscess has formed, an annular constriction, which marks the site of the primary growth often reveals the nature of the problem and the need to resect the lymphatic glands draining the area. Immediate resection should then be undertaken or the growth removed within a month if a colostomy is performed.

A few patients will be unfit to withstand major surgery; those with diverticulitis may live many years in comfort with a colostomy. Sometimes, they improve as the infection settles and become well enough to tolerate resection and later closure of the colostomy.

Finally, it should be remembered that constipation, especially in the very old, may be the cause of fatal obstruction (Rao and Katarla, 1967). This is another good reason for ensuring that the stools are soft and easily passed in every patient.

Chapter 18

Complicated Diverticular Disease: Haemorrhage

This complication of colonic diverticula was first described in 1903 by Koch (Dunning, 1963) and later by de Quervain (1927). Unfortunately, Telling and Gruner (1917) believed that bleeding was almost unknown in diverticulosis and this erroneous attitude has persisted so that, even today, there are those who are reluctant to diagnose diverticular disease as the source of rectal bleeding. It is only in the last 25 years that haemorrhage from diverticulosis has attracted much attention, despite the fact that Morton (1946) recorded that bleeding was the presenting symptom in 21·6% of 111 patients, and Ulin and his colleagues (1959) reported a total of 50 examples of massive haemorrhage from diverticula.

The anatomical basis of haemorrhage from diverticulosis was investigated by Noer (1955) who injected the colonic blood vessels with coloured latex and demonstrated their intimate relationship with the mucosal sacs. He collected 2,896 cases in which haemorrhage occurred in no less than 11% and since that time bleeding from colonic diverticula has become a recognized problem in clinical surgery. The magnitude of this problem has not been defined accurately. Its incidence varies from as low as 5% (Healey and Pfeffer, 1965) to up to 40% in some series, and it would be fair to say that about 30% of those known to have colonic diverticula bleed at some time or another.

THE PATHOGENESIS OF BLEEDING IN DIVERTICULOSIS

This is still a matter for debate. Noer (1959) published beautiful photographs which showed that quite large vessels surround the mucosal sacs and which make it easy to understand how serious bleeding could occur once the integrity of these vessels has been breached, but the trigger mechanism that initiates the bleeding process in but a few of thousands of diverticula, has not been identified with certainty. It is tempting to blame local diverticulitis for necrosis of the vessels and the subsequent brisk haemorrhage. Pyogenic granulation tissue has been found in diverticula that have bled, Olsen (1968), but this abnormality is usually the source of only mild bleeding (Dunning, 1963). Clinically, signs of diverticulitis, such as fever, leucocytosis and local tenderness are noticeably absent in patients with recurrent episodes of bleeding, and even in those whose lives are endangered by massive exsanguinating haemorrhage. Hence there is little evidence with which to incriminate infection as the cause of this complication (Heald & Ray, 1971).

Bleeding occurs in diverticulosis without any preceding constitutional upset or signs of true diverticulitis. This state of affairs can be compared with bleeding from jejunal diverticula, which happens in a part of the bowel whose contents are sterile and which is not prone to inflammation.

Hence local mechanical trauma has been blamed for bleeding. The friction of a faecolith may damage a vessel but one would expect haemorrhage to be commoner if this were a common cause. Inversion of diverticula has been recorded and such an event would be expected to damage any vessel that was adherent to the mucosal sac. Young and Howorth (1954), reported that an inverted diverticulum had acted like a polyp and had initiated intussusception of the splenic flexure. They believed that the resultant trauma could cause local vessels to bleed. Others believe that infection localized to the mouths of diverticula is responsible for bleeding (Quinn, 1961; Dunning, 1963). Adam Smith (1974, personal communication) suggested that diverticula which are still reducible might herniate only at intervals and, in so doing, damage blood vessels in their immediate vicinity, much in the same way as the strangulation of an inguinal hernia may obstruct the blood supply of the gut. However, it is fair to say that if these were the main factors responsible for haemorrhage in diverticular disease, this complication would be expected to be seen much more frequently in this very common disease.

Another factor is worthy of consideration, namely the effect of the increasing incidence of atherosclerosis in the Western world. Bleeding in diverticulosis has only attracted attention since the 1950s. Diverticulitis was only recognized as a cause of death by the Registrar General of England and Wales in 1923 and coronary artery disease was accredited the same distinction only in 1926. It is therefore reasonable to take the view that bleeding in diverticular disease is comparable to cerebral haemorrhage, because in both conditions bleeding runs from a diseased artery which is ill-supported by its surrounding tissues. Like cerebro-vascular accidents, haemorrhage in diverticulitis is seen most commonly in elderly hypertensive patients and is rare below the age of 50 (Olsen, 1968); Earley (1959) recorded that no less than 18 of his 32 patients suffered from arterial disease, and ischaemic heart disease is associated epidemiologically with diverticulosis (Trowell, Painter and Burkitt, 1974). Arteriosclerosis is commoner in patients with diabetes which is also associated with diverticulitis (Schowengerdt *et al.*, 1969). All these three degenerative diseases are extremely prevalent in the industrial nations of the West and may be caused by the over-refining of carbohydrates (Cleave, Campbell & Painter, 1969). Both diverticular disease and arteriosclerosis may be caused, at least in part, by a deficiency of dietary fibre (Trowell, Painter & Burkitt, 1974). Hence it is not surprising that the arteries supplying the colon are arteriosclerotic in most patients with diverticular disease and so are unable to withstand the effects of infection or trauma. It is possible that they may be injured by the abnormally high intracolonic pressures that cause diverticulosis, but as yet there is no proof of this.

CLINICAL PRESENTATION

Haemorrhage due to diverticulosis may be mild, moderate or severe.

Mild Haemorrhage

The majority of cases fall into this group, although Ramanath and Hinshaw (1971) found that approximately one third of their patients fell into each group. The average patient is elderly, probably hypertensive, and passes recognizable blood in small amounts, independent of defaecation. The amount of blood lost has no effect on the patient's general condition and bleeding ceases spontaneously with bed rest and sedation. Recurrent episodes of such bleeding, some of which pass unnoticed by the patient, may lead to severe anaemia.

The diagnosis is made by exclusion and the demonstration of colonic diverticula. The colon must be examined by sigmoid-oscopy, barium enema and by colonoscopy if this is available. The presence of any bleeding diathesis must be excluded. *Such bleeding must be assumed to be caused by a carcinoma of the colon or rectum until proved otherwise.*

The treatment of mild haemorrhage consists of rest in bed and sedation. Both single and multiple episodes of bleeding may lead to anaemia which must be corrected by giving iron and vitamin C and by transfusion if necessary. Elderly hyper-tensive patients do not tolerate anaemia well. After their recovery patients should be placed on a high fibre diet, which will relieve symptoms in most cases, but which does not prevent further episodes of haemorrhage. The author has performed one left hemicolectomy and one subtotal colectomy for bleeding in patients who had taken bran for over a year and who were otherwise symptom free.

Moderate Haemorrhage

Bleeding begins suddenly and usually without previous symptoms. The patient experiences an unexpected call to stool which may be preceded by slight colic in the left iliac fossa or by a feeling of distension, or may be unheralded by any symptoms. Red or maroon blood is passed per rectum in copious amounts. There is no fever, leucocytosis or clinical evidence of diverticulitis. Bleeding may stop as dramatically as it began or may continue until several pints have been lost, sometimes giving rise to diarrhoea. The degree of shock will depend on the rate at which blood is lost. Some patients show no sign of shock even when they are profoundly anaemic because they have adapted to the effects of small but recurrent haemorrhages.

Treatment consists of rest, sedation and careful observation. The blood should be examined for its coagulability and haemo-globin content. Blood transfusion may be necessary especially in the elderly and hypertensive who do not tolerate haemorrhage well. Many old patients are deficient of vitamins and this should be corrected; vitamin C especially should be given. Calcium gluconate and vitamin K have also been administered by many surgeons including the author despite the lack of any evidence that they are of immediate benefit.

As soon as the patient's condition permits, the diagnosis is established by the usual investigations and the presence of malignant disease is ruled out. The patient is then put on a high residue diet with supplements of vitamins and iron as required. The possible co-existence of conditions such as diabetes mellitus and hypertension must always be borne in mind and the patient placed under the care of a physician if these disorders are present.

Severe Haemorrhage

Sudden severe haemorrhage may occur without warning in patients who have diverticulosis even though there is no evidence that they are suffering from diverticulitis. Bleeding may be so rapid that the patient becomes exsanguinated. This can be extremely dangerous as arteriosclerosis is common in the age group concerned so that many patients are unable to compensate for blood loss and must be transfused as a matter of urgency if they are to survive. Fortunately, this is the least common form of haemorrhage, and usually stops spontaneously. Fraenkel (1954) reviewed 15 cases of severe bleeding admitted to the Radcliffe Infirmary, Oxford, between 1946 and 1951. He quoted the dictum of D. C. Corry, surgeon to that hospital, namely that 'if a middle aged or elderly patient, apparently in good health, has a sudden unexpected and alarmingly profuse rectal haemorrhage of perhaps several pints, full investigation is likely to reveal diverticulosis of the colon and the bleeding is unlikely to continue'.

This statement is true, in the main, as 81 % of patients recover without operative intervention (Ramanath and Hinshaw, 1971). Unfortunately, bleeding may continue and it is these patients who present a difficult problem. Surgeons are reluctant to operate knowing that bleeding usually stops and also because it is so difficult to localize the site of bleeding before or even at laparotomy. This is made more difficult by the fact that patients with extensive diverticulosis are about eight times more likely to have a massive haemorrhage; and also because bleeding from the right half of the colon is much more frequent than would be expected in a predominantly left-sided disease. Consequently surgeons tend to interfere too late in cases of unrelenting haemorrhage (Hoare, 1970, Quinn, 1961; Lewis and Schnug, 1972).

Investigations

The condition of the patient may limit the investigations that can be performed. The blood must be examined not only to determine its haemoglobin content but to ensure that coagulation is normal. A naso-gastric tube should be passed to see if the stomach contains blood. The absence of blood rules out bleeding from a peptic ulcer. Blood passed per rectum was dark and tarry in 42 out of 100 cases (Ramanath and Hinshaw, 1971), however, when bleeding is brisk the colour changes to maroon or bright red. The amount of blood lost may be greater than that passed per rectum as the colon can contain several pints of blood. This possibility should be borne in mind when the patient's condition is worse than would be expected from the apparent blood loss.

The replacement of blood by transfusion is a matter of urgency, Patients in this age group who are hypertensive have rigid vascular trees and do not tolerate hypotension well. The rate of blood loss is as important a factor as the amount lost and so it is wise to have blood cross matched even before transfusion is necessary so as to anticipate a sudden increase in the rate of haemorrhage.

If possible, barium studies should be performed in an attempt to find the cause and site of the bleeding. Although sigmoidoscopy has been known to reveal a bleeding diverticulum, this is very rare, and this investigation is seldom helpful.

Arteriography has a place in the diagnosis and the treatment of bleeding in diverticulosis. Lewis and Schnug (1972) could find recorded only 31 cases of the precise localization of the point of bleeding in the literature and 13 of these had been demonstrated by angiography. Their technique is as follows. Once the patient's condition permits, selective mesenteric angiography is carried out and contrast material which escapes from the bleeding vessel can be seen pooling in the lumen of the colon. After localization, the offending vessel is perfused with epinephrine solutions at a rate of 20 ml. per minute for 15 minutes. If a repeat angiogram shows no further bleeding, the catheter is left in place and the patient returned to the ward. A repeat angiogram is performed next day and if bleeding has ceased, the catheter is removed. Their plan of management consists of (1) intubation of the stomach, (2) blood transfusion to stabilize the patient's condition, (3) blood coagulation studies, (4) sigmoidoscopy, (5) angiography and the administration of vasoconstrictors, (6) barium enema and finally, surgery if this proves to be necessary.

They undertake angiography only if the patient requires more than three units of blood in 24 hours and when bleeding continues for 36 hours, and consider that selective angiography is indicated if bleeding stops but then restarts. Angiography is safe and the giving of vasoconstrictors has proved effective, but it is essential that this investigation is carried out while the patient is bleeding so that contrast material will escape into the colon. Bleeding rates as low as 0·5 ml./minute can be detected by this method. More massive haemorrhage almost ensures that the bleeding point will be identified. Blood can be transfused while selective catheterization of the mesenteric vessels is taking place and the whole procedure can be carried out in less than one hour by an experienced radiologist.

If vasoconstrictors fail to stop the bleeding, a barium enema is given. This is justified as frequently haemorrhage from diverticula ceases after a barium enema. The reason for this is not clear. If this is not effective, surgery is indicated with the surgeon having the advantage of knowing which part of the colon to resect. Needless to say, this technique represents a great advance in dealing with this uncommon emergency, but it can only be used in hospitals who have the facilities and staff to give this service by both day and night.

THE INDICATIONS FOR SURGERY

Laparotomy must be performed when conservative means fail and the patient's life is in danger. This is a matter of clinical judgement. Once it seems certain that bleeding is of colonic origin and not due to carcinoma, Crohn's disease or ulcerative colitis, the decision to operate must be made even if the site of the bleeding has not been determined. As with patients who are bleeding from peptic ulceration, the mortality rises if operation is delayed until 10 or 14 pints of blood have been given. Ramanath and Hinshaw (1971) noted that two patients given an average of 14,000 ml. of blood both died, and others have noted that the prognosis following a second massive hamorrhage is worse. Hence it is best to operate while the patient's condition is still good.

(a) Localization of the bleeding point at Laparotomy

At operation the colon may be full of blood and the source of bleeding is seldom apparent. Weingarten, Venet and Victor (1959) adopted the following method of finding the bleeding vessel. The colon is occluded by light clamps at the hepatic and splenic flexure. A colotomy is made in the sigmoid and the left colon evacuated of blood. If it refills, then a left hemicolectomy is performed unless the bleeding vessel can be identified and sutured. If the left colon does not refill the caecum is opened and the procedure is repeated. Finally, the transverse colon is opened if necessary. If the vessel is seen bleeding it can be sutured or, if not, the part of the colon that refills with blood is excised. Usually an end to end anastomosis is made at once, but if the patient's condition does not permit this, continuity of the bowel may be restored at a later operation.

(b) 'Blind' Hemicolectomy

If this procedure is not carried out, the surgeon has the choice of excising that part of the colon that bears diverticula in the hope of removing the bleeding vessel or of performing a subtotal colectomy with ileo-rectal anastomosis. At first sight, it seems reasonable to perform a left hemicolectomy if the diverticula are limited to this side of the colon, but this may be followed by a recurrence of bleeding if this originated in the right half of the colon. Massive haemorrhage requiring 12 pints of blood has complicated the presence of a caecal diverticulum (Taylor, 1966) and so 'blind' hemicolectomy is not to be recommended.

(c) The Place of Diversionary Colostomy

Dunning (1963) advocated the use of a right transverse colostomy when bleeding from diverticular disease did not respond to conservative treatment, providing no carcinoma was present. He thought that emergency resection should be avoided as it had a high mortality. It is difficult to understand how diversion of the faecal stream would help to stop bleeding and the author believes that the successful use of this manoeuvre could be explained quite easily by coincidence especially when it is remembered that even massive haemorrhage may cease spontaneously. Only when a patient is too critically ill to withstand resection or subtotal colectomy should a colostomy or an ileostomy be fashioned, but there is no certainty that either manoeuvre will arrest the haemorrhage (Earley, 1959; Quinn, 1961).

(d) Ligation of Bleeding Vessel and Exteriorization of the Opened loop of Colon

If the site of bleeding is known before operation or found at laparotomy the offending vessel should be ligated. This is simple and effective, but closure of the colotomy may be time consuming and it may be easier to exteriorize the opened loop of colon together with the ligated vessel. This procedure is quick and restoration of the bowel's continuity may be undertaken later when the patient is no longer exsanguinated.

(e) Subtotal colectomy

Massive unrelenting haemorrhage leading to laparotomy can be arrested by resection of the entire colon with ileorectal anastomosis. The anastomosis may be delayed and undertaken at a second operation, but the removal of all the diverticula will, if the diagnosis is correct, prevent further blood loss. Total abdominal colectomy appears to have been feared quite needlessly. In the absence of a carcinoma, no dissection of the mesocolon and lymph nodes is necessary and the operation can be accomplished rapidly. Moreover an ileorectal anastomosis can be fashioned without tension, and will be subjected only to the passage of semi-liquid contents post-operatively. Patients, treated by subtotal colectomy, pass about three stools a day and do not suffer from any disability. They cannot contract carcinoma of the colon in the future (Ramanath and Hinshaw, 1971; Heald and Ray, 1971).

(f) Prophylactic Resection to Prevent Recurrent Haemorrhage

Some authors have recommended that elective subtotal colectomy should be carried out to prevent subsequent bleeding after a single episode of major haemorrhage. This is not justified as it has been estimated that only from 10% to 25% bleed at a later date (Lewis and Schnug, 1972). Recurrent episodes of bleeding which produce profound anaemia are an indication for resection of all the colon that bears diverticula and if necessary, subtotal colectomy. The author performed a total colectomy for recurrent anaemia and the patient has remained well for seven years. The temptation to preserve the caecum and anastomose it to the rectum must be resisted as the caecum may be the site of diverticulosis or of an angioma,

CONCLUSION

Bleeding which may be severe occurs in diverticulosis. In the great majority of patients, it stops with bed rest and transfusion if this becomes necessary. The few that require surgery should be operated on before their condition deteriorates. If it is possible to demonstrate the site of bleeding by pre-operative angiography or at operation, ligation of the offending vessel or local resection is all that is required. If the site of bleeding is not known, emergency subtotal colectomy with, or without, immediate anastomosis is the procedure of choice. Prophylactic resection is indicated if recurrent episodes of bleeding lead to profound anaemia.

Chapter 19

Diverticular Disease of the Caecum, Ascending and Transverse Colon

Diverticulitis of the caecum, ascending and transverse colon may be part of a generalized disease process that involves the whole of the large bowel down to and sometimes including even the rectum. This pattern is common in the Western nations but it has been realized recently that the right half of the colon may be affected by the disease while the left side of the colon is normal more often than had been thought previously. In particular, diverticulosis is found in the caecum and ascending colon in certain Eastern countries more often than in the West and this variety of the disease most commonly afflicts younger patients in their middle 40s.

Caecal diverticulitis treated by diverticulectomy was described by Potier (1912) and, by 1937, Bennett-Jones could collect only 20 cases from the literature. Since then, diverticula of the caecum and ascending colon have been described with increasing frequency. Their aetiology is still unknown and no systematic studies of the pressures within the caecum and ascending colon have been made. Muscle thickening does not precede the appearance of diverticula in this part of the large bowel as it does in the sigmoid, and this suggests that right-sided diverticulosis is a different disease. True diverticula of the caecum with complete muscular coats have been described but they must be extremely rare. For practical purposes, diverticula of the caecum and proximal colon are acquired herniations.

INCIDENCE OF DIVERTICULOSIS AND DIVERTICULITIS OF THE ASCENDING COLON AND CAECUM

(1) IN THE WESTERN COUNTRIES

Miangolarra (1961) studied 758 patients with diverticulosis in New Orleans. The right half of the colon was affected in 231

(30%) patients and in 109 (14%) diverticulosis was present on the right half of the colon while its left half was normal. This variety of diverticula tend to give rise to diverticulitis around the age of 40 which, on average, is about 20 years before left-sided diverticula cause symptoms. In coloured citizens of New Orleans, diverticula are restricted to the caecum and ascending colon in over 20% of patients. This is very different from the Australian scene, where Hughes (1969) found that diverticulosis affected the sigmoid in 95% of cases and in only 5% was the caecum alone diseased. He reported that caecal diverticula could be present without any thickening of the sigmoid musculature. These observations support the view that caecal diverticula are caused by local factors independent of those that lead to diverticular disease of the sigmoid. 'Solitary' diverticula of the caecum have been described; these have been found at laparotomy but if barium studies are performed later they are usually shown to be only one of many caecal diverticula (Schapira *et al.*, 1958).

(2) IN EASTERN COUNTRIES

The distribution of diverticula around the colon differs in some Eastern countries from the pattern which is so well known in the West. The reason for this is unknown. The disease was rare in Japan until recently but between 1967 and 1971, 131 cases of diverticulosis were demonstrated in 1,987 patients at the Tokyo Women's Hospital, an incidence of 6·6%. Men were three times as prone to the condition as women; no less than 22·2% of males over 70 years old had diverticula. This sex ratio differs from that seen in the West but an even more striking difference is that in 87 of the 131 cases, the caecum and ascending colon bore diverticula, an incidence of 67% (Yazawa, 1973).

In Hawaii, where immigrant Japanese and their descendants have adopted American eating habits since the attack on Pearl Harbor in 1941 (Stemmerman, personal communication, 1973), diverticulosis affects Americans of Japanese stock extremely frequently but the right side of their colons is diseased much more often than that of their Caucasian compatriots. Chang (1965) analysed 414 cases of diverticulitis admitted to three Hawaiian hospitals between 1956 and 1962. Among these were a 21-year-old Japanese male with caecal diverticulitis and a Caucasian woman of 87 with sigmoid diverticulitis. No less than 261 (79·3%) of 329 cases of left-sided diverticulitis were seen in

Caucasians; only 10·6% occurred in Japanese, 5% in Chinese and the remaining few were found in Philippinos, Hawaiians and Koreans. By contrast, 53 (62·3%) of 85 cases of right-sided diverticulitis occurred in Japanese and only 14 (16·4%) were seen in Caucasians.

Chang noted that patients with diverticulitis of the right colon had an average age of 44·5 years, which is about 20 years earlier than the average age at which patients with left-sided diverticulitis are admitted to hospital. He considered that the effects of diet on the distribution of diverticula in Hawaiian Japanese was worthy of study in order to see if the prevalence and the presentation of the disease altered in the second and third generation Japanese who had been reared as Americans and subjected to the effects of a Western diet since birth.

Diverticular disease is seen in the left half of the colon in 95% of Caucasians in Hawaii, a pattern essentially similar to that seen in the continental United States and Europe, whereas 60% of diverticulitis in Hawaiian Japanese is found in the caecum and ascending colon. No muscle thickening accompanies this latter form of the disease which suggests that it may have a separate aetiology (Peck *et al.*, 1968). These findings have been confirmed by Stemmerman (1970) and by Stemmerman and Yatani (1973).

In Hawaian Japanese, right-sided diverticula disease appears in a younger age group while the incidence of both the right- and left-sided forms of the disease increase in frequency up to the eighth decade. After 80 years, diverticular disease becomes less prevalent in Japanese; this may be due to the fact that the oldest Japanese immigrants did not adopt Western eating habits until the Second World War, so that those over 80 years old were not subjected to this environmental influence in the first half of their lives.

However, this does not account for the tendency of diverticulosis to affect the right half of the colon in Japanese, Chinese, Hawaiians, Philippinos and Koreans because even in younger Hawaiian Japanese, 50% of diverticula are found in the right half of the colon and only 40% on the left (Stemmerman and Yatani, 1973). This pattern is the opposite of that seen in Europe, North America and Australasia. The reason for this is not known but it suggests that there are at least two varieties of diverticular disease or that a factor related to race is operating.

Clinical Features

Diverticula of the caecum, ascending and transverse colon which are not inflamed usually cause no symptoms. Their presence is discovered incidentally by barium studies and they only become a clinical problem if they become infected or bleed.

Whether uninflamed diverticula produce symptoms is still unknown. Miangolarra (1961) reported that only 26 of 109 patients with right-sided diverticula complained of symptoms. Patients with diverticula confined to the caecum and ascending colon may suffer recurrent episodes of mild abdominal pain at regular intervals. They may be investigated for peptic ulceration, biliary disease or appendicular colic and be treated by appendicectomy or cholecystectomy. The bowel habit is not changed as in the case of sigmoid diverticular disease but sometimes patients have attacks of diarrhoea. Whether these symptoms are caused by the diverticula is still uncertain, but occasionally the right colon has been resected for diverticular disease accompanied by recurrent pain.

If diverticula in this region are found, and the presence of a co-existing carcinoma has been ruled out, no treatment is necessary. There is no evidence as yet that a high-fibre diet is of benefit. However, pain in the right iliac fossa often accompanies constipation and so it is the author's practice to prescribe bran. This may relieve discomfort in the right side of the abdomen but whether this was caused by the diverticula is still a matter for speculation (Schapiro *et al.*, 1958; Miangolarra, 1961).

ACUTE DIVERTICULITIS

Acute diverticulitis of the caecum and ascending colon is usually indistinguishable clinically from acute appendicitis. If a mass is palpable, the differential diagnosis includes an appendix abscess, Crohn's disease, carcinoma or disease of the Fallopian tubes; Tagart (1953) would add 'acute phlegmonous caecitis' to this but this may be only another manifestation of caecal diverticulitis.

Examination reveals tenderness in the right iliac fossa or right upper quadrant of the abdomen. Tenderness may be elicited on the right side by the finger on rectal examination. A palpable mass may be present if an abscess has formed. Rupture of an inflamed diverticulum may give rise to peritonitis; the treatment of this complication has been discussed in Chapter 15.

Fever is not marked and the white cell count is usually raised. Nausea and vomiting occur less frequently than in acute appendicitis. The diagnosis is seldom made pre-operatively in Europe and the U.S.A., but diverticulitis is often suspected when Hawaiian Japanese are admitted with acute abdominal pain on the right side. In one series of 58 cases requiring surgery, a diagnosis of acute appendicitis was made no less than 54 times (Fairbank and Rob, 1947; Sanderson and Madigan, 1954; Schapiro *et al.*, 1958; Miangolarra, 1961; Peck *et al.*, 1968).

SURGICAL TREATMENT OF ACUTE DIVERTICULITIS OF THE CAECUM AND ASCENDING COLON

Most patients will be operated upon in the belief that they are suffering from acute appendicitis. If a grid-iron incision is made, this will be adequate if a solitary inflamed diverticulum is found or if an abscess has to be drained, but if this incision gives insufficient access, it should be closed and the abdomen opened through a right paramedian incision.

Once it is obvious that the operator is not dealing with acute appendicitis, the situation must be reassessed carefully. Every effort must be made to exclude the presence of a carcinoma. This may be impossible especially if an abscess has formed.

An inflamed single diverticulum may be excised and the caecum closed or the diverticulum may be invaginated with a purse-string suture (Reid, 1951). An abscess should be drained and the patient investigated by barium enema after recovering from the emergency operation.

If the inflammatory process has involved part of the caecal wall and the lymph glands are enlarged, it may be impossible to be sure whether a carcinoma is present or not. In these circumstances, an immediate right hemicolectomy should be performed.

If a large abscess has formed, when dealing with poor risk patients, surgery should be limited to closing any perforation and drainage. The true pathology can be determined later and if carcinoma is suspected, a right hemicolectomy must be performed as soon as possible. Alternatively, a local mass can be resected by the Paul-Mickulicz technique. Local excision of the terminal ileum and caecum may be necessary if the inflammatory process has obstructed the small gut (Peck *et al.*, 1968).

Schapiro and his colleagues (1958) advise against emergency resection in the presence of infection and prefer to exteriorize the diseased bowel. However, any fears they have regarding the safety of emergency resection of the right colon are unfounded. Emergency right hemicolectomy carries little risk as the result-ant ileo-colic anastomosis, unlike one made in the sigmoid, can be made without tension and only has to cope with fluid con-tents and so can be accomplished with a very low morbidity. The patient is thus cured with one operation. If this is not pos-sible and the slightest doubt as to the diagnosis exists, barium studies must be performed post-operatively supplemented by colonoscopy if the diagnosis is still uncertain.

HAEMORRHAGE FROM THE RIGHT HALF OF THE COLON

A high proportion of those with diverticulosis of the caecum and ascending colon pass occult blood, have frank melaena or suffer a massive haemorrhage. Miangolarra (1961) considered that melaena was an 'outstanding symptom' which occurred in 47% of his series of diverticulosis restricted to the right half of the colon. Twenty-two of these required transfusion, 14 of them responded to blood replacement and eight, aged 47 to 81 years old, were treated by emergency surgery. This consisted of a right hemicolectomy in most cases or subtotal colectomy if the trans-verse colon was affected. In one patient operated upon for bleeding, both diverticulosis and carcinoma existed together. The difficulty of determining the true pathology even after opening a caecum that is full of blood is another argument in favour of emergency right hemicolectomy. Taylor (1966) described the passage of bright red blood per rectum from an ulcer adjacent to the appendix. When palpation showed it to have a hard edge, a right hemicolectomy was carried out that was followed by a rapid improvement in the patient's blood pressure. Histological examination revealed that the bleeding was from a diverticulum.

DIVERTICULOSIS OF THE TRANSVERSE COLON

Diverticula in the transverse colon may bleed or perforate like diverticula elsewhere but on rare occasions they perforate and a mass forms whose nature is uncertain at laparotomy. Lockhart-Mummery (1949) operated on a woman who was thought to have acute appendicitis only to find a tumour the size of a small hen's egg six inches distal to the hepatic flexure. This was hard and did not appear to be of inflammatory origin. It was resected by the Paul-Mickulicz technique and found to be caused by the perforation of a diverticulum 2 cm. in depth. He was only able to find another example of diverticulitis in the transverse colon, namely, that described by Thompson and Fox (1944) in a man of 35.

Since then, Rowlands (1957) has reported another case and Sagar (1973) has published what is probably the first account of a giant diverticulum of the transverse colon. Sagan's patient was a woman of 75 with pain but who was otherwise well. A tender swelling 15–20 cm. in diameter was present in the left upper quadrant and this moved with respiration. A barium enema showed diverticulosis of the sigmoid and descending colon and a large solitary diverticulum arising from the superior margin of the transverse colon. This was resected successfully and found to be a giant diverticulum filled with faeces and gas, and covered with omentum. Eleven such giant diverticula have been described in the descending and sigmoid colon but a survey of the literature revealed no report of one situated in the transverse colon. It has been suggested that they are caused by intermittent occlusion of the neck of the diverticulum trapping gas under high pressure or by distension caused by gas-forming micro-organisms.

Chapter 20

Reilly's Operation of Sigmoid Myotomy

'When in doubt, take it out' is a catch phrase that has been known to generations of surgeons, but its validity should be questioned at regular intervals. Resection has been the mainstay of the surgical treatment of diverticulitis and also of painful diverticular disease for 30 years because it offered the only hope of curing these two manifestations of the disease; but just as partial gastrectomy for duodenal ulceration yielded pride of place to vagotomy, it is possible that resection of the sigmoid colon may be replaced on occasions by Reilly's operation of sigmoid myotomy.

Reilly (1964, 1966, 1969, 1971) realized that there was often little fibrosis and no ulceration to be found in resected sigmoid colons and that the main abnormality was often a well-demarcated stricture caused by thickening of the muscle coat with infolding of the inter-haustral folds and of the mucosa. It seemed to him a pity to resect this bowel if its lumen could be widened and to perform what is often a difficult anastomosis. Therefore, in 1961, he considered the operation of sigmoid myotomy; this was before the work of Morson (1963) and Slack (1962) had been published.

OPERATIVE TECHNIQUE

I am indebted to Mr Michael Reilly of Plymouth for the following description of the procedure which he has made popular.

'The appearances of the muscle in specimens resected for diverticular disease are reminiscent of the appearances of the pyloric muscle in congenital pyloric hypertrophy. The muscle, especially the circular muscle, is thickened, pale and oedematous and can be divided quite easily. It was found that the circular muscle can be split longitudinally right down to the mucosa and it seemed feasible that this would be equally simple to do in a living patient. This would avoid the risks of wide resection of the colon in diverticular disease. As contemporary teaching maintained that the condition was progressive and might affect the whole of the left colon, it was the practice to remove a considerable length of the colon. This necessitated wide mobilization of the colon and sometimes anastomosis of the transverse colon to the upper rectum. If resection was more limited, it was not necessarily technically easier because the sigmoid mesocolon was often thickened and shortened due to fatty infiltration and fibrosis due to past inflammation and lymphangitis. Anastomoses made under tension were liable to leak or break down leading to abscess and fistula formation or to peritonitis and death. These complications still occur even with modern antibiotics and supportive therapy.

As the inflammation of diverticulitis is often confined to one or more diverticula outside the colonic wall, it seemed illogical to resect a piece of bowel whose mucosa appeared normal and whose muscle was only thickened. It seemed more sensible to leave the bowel 'in situ' and to divide the muscle coat longitudinally, thus relieving the constriction of the lumen and lessening the intracolonic pressure so as to lessen the likelihood of perforation.

The longitudinal muscle of the colon is gathered into three bands or taeniae, one at the mesocolic attachment, while the other two are placed laterally between which a strip of bowel wall is thrown into undulating folds. These represent the haustra which are covered only by peritoneum and a thin layer of circular muscle. By contrast, the rectum is covered uniformly by a complete layer of longitudinal muscle. This longitudinal muscle becomes separated into taeniae an inch or two above the rectosigmoid junction. In diverticular disease, not only is the circular muscle thickened but the longitudinal muscle is shortened so that the two antimesocolic taeniae are thicker and widened until they lie almost side by side being separated by only a small slit instead of a wide band of circular muscle. An incision made in the strict antimesocolic line starting over the recto-sigmoid junction and prolonged upwards will first pass between the fibres of an unbroken sheet of longitudinal muscle and then divide the underlying circular fibres down to the submucosa. As this incision is continued upwards, it will incise the slit between the taeniae.

When the operation was first performed this was not appreciated and it was thought that the incision was through a taenia. The present practice is to make the incision between the approximated taeniae and to prolong it upwards through the thickened part of the sigmoid and descending colon until the bowel appears and feels to be normal. Hence, the incision may be 1 in. to 15 in. in length. Where the bowel becomes relatively normal, the taeniae diverge and the incision can be continued upwards for another one or two inches (Fig. 61).

In practice, it has been found difficult to incise the undulating circular muscle between the taeniae without perforating the mucosa and so the incision is placed in one of the mesocolic taeniae that is nearest to the 'mid-line'. This lessens the likelihood of dividing submucous blood vessels of any size as the segmental blood vessels are smallest at this point of the colon's circumference, having given off their lateral branches. Hence, the midline incision is relatively bloodless and, with care, no blood vessels are divided. If a vessel is cut, no cautery nor ligature should be applied as this may cause necrosis and later perforation. It is best not to be too thorough and not to denude the bulging mucosa of every transverse strand of tissue. When in doubt it is better to leave a few fibres uncut and to turn one's attention to deepening another part of the incision. The incision is started with a scalpel from below up and then widened from above downwards with the scissors. When these fibres are inspected again after an interval, it will be found that most of the cut oedematous circular muscle fibres have retracted, allowing the mucosa to bulge through the longitudinal incision. Any obvious bundles of circular fibres may then be more easily recognized and divided. Isolated strands may be blood vessels. They should not be divided: if they are vessels they are supplying the mucosa, and being elastic do not constrict the lumen. If they are single muscle strands, not bundles, their constricting power is negligible. Any bleeding should be controlled by a damp swab. This is invariably effective. The use of adrenalin is unnecessary and diathermy may perforate the mucosa.

Sigmoid myotomy is surprisingly easy if performed with care and patience. It is most important to mobilize the sigmoid colon by dividing its secondary attachments to the left wall of the pelvis so that it becomes a mid-line organ again. The peritoneum is divided laterally in a bloodless plane and then the sigmoid colon

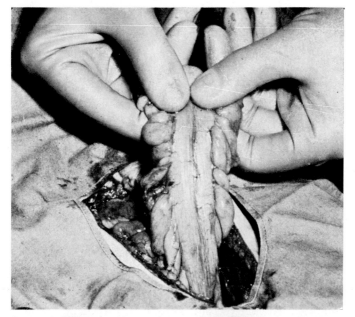

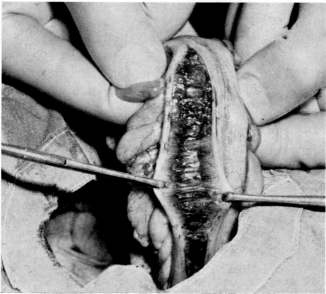

Fig. 61a. Shows sigmoid colon mobilized so that it is straight. This is an essential manoeuvre as it enables the operator to make a straight incision.

Fig 61b. Shows the same sigmoid with most of the circular muscle divided. Glistening mucosa can be seen bulging between a few remaining circular muscle bundles. These become more obvious when cut oedematous muscle has slowly retracted. They can then be easily divided. There is no need to cut every single transverse strand of tissue. Some strands may be blood vessels. Too much thoroughness may lead to bleeding. This is easily controlled by a wet swab, but a denuded mucosa may perforate later.

can be held straight by pulling it taut from the recto-sigmoid junction. This makes it easier to keep the incision straight and in the bloodless 'mid-line' and to prolong it below the recto-sigmoid junction. This is an essential part of the operation as it is here that there is a physiological sphincter which controls the passage of faeces from the colon into the rectum. It is 'this 'sphincter' which is so familiar to sigmoidoscopists and which often prevents the passage of the instrument beyond 15 cm. from the anus. This is usually attributed to 'spasm' and is well known to radiologists who often have difficulty in getting barium to pass this point. The structure of this sphincter has not been described and it is more of a physiological than an anatomical sphincter. Hughes (1969) has recently described the presence of lateral crescentic folds of circular muscle which may act partly as a sphincter and partly as a sling which pulls the left wall of the recto-sigmoid across to the right, angulating the junction of the sigmoid with the rectum. Thus, a shelf is formed which will hold up the larger masses of faeces, if not small scybala and liquid stools.

Although myotomy does not divide these lateral crescents of muscle, it enlarges the lumen and possibly prevents the forces which make the mechanism described by Hughes effective.

The raw area formed by the incision need not be covered by peritoneum as described by Daniels (1969) and there is no need to insert a drain if the mucosa is intact. If the mucosa is perforated inadvertently, it is usually obvious and it is not necessary to perform the tests which have been advocated by some authors. One such test is to fill the pelvis with saline or saline mixed with Cetavlon and then to inflate the rectum with air. The procedure is similar to that used to detect punctures in an inner tube as bubbles will escape from a perforation. If Cetavlon has been used, iridescent bubbles will add interest to the procedure as they float round the operating theatre!

If the mucosa has been accidentally perforated, all that is necessary is to suture it with fine catgut and to close the abdomen with a pelvic drain. A defunctioning colostomy should only be necessary if a major perforation or other pathology such as pericolic abscess threaten the integrity of the bowel. If the mucosa has not been perforated, the colon is simply replaced in the pelvis with the myotomy incision turned towards the left lateral wall of the pelvis.

On only one occasion, in nearly one hundred cases has this technique resulted in complications. In this patient, a short mesocolon made it impossible to ensure that the raw area was in contact with the pelvic wall and a loop of small bowel became adherent causing obstruction postoperatively. This necessitated a second operation some days later.

Mr Reilly has performed nearly a hundred operations. Three quarters of these patients required surgery for uncomplicated diverticular disease causing symptoms of sufficient severity to be a nuisance and a potential danger. Some had suffered pain for years and others had been admitted to hospital for medical treatment on more than one occasion. The remaining one quarter had diverticular disease complicated by pelvic abscess, with or without obstruction, vesico-colic or other fistula. Such problems required staged procedures. Usually, a preliminary colostomy was followed by the definitive operation and the colostomy was closed a few weeks later. If all signs of acute inflammation have disappeared, the definitive operation may be that of myotomy if the bowel can be mobilized and inspected. If local abscesses or fistula persist, it is better to resect the most affected part of the sigmoid and to anastomose with a myotomy above or below it, or both if necessary. This combination of local resection and myotomy makes it unnecessary to resect as much colon as has been necessary in the past so that mobilization of the splenic flexure and the opening up of retroperitoneal tissue planes is avoided.

One word of warning. Resection may be indicated instead of myotomy. It is unfortunate that early in the series satisfactory results were obtained when treating fistula by myotomy. This led to a false feeling of confidence until one chronic fistula which had been oversewn broke down and caused further complications. The myotomy was intact and healing well but it appeared that fibrosis consequent upon the chronicity of the fistula had prevented it healing. In such a case, resection with or without myotomy is indicated.

At first, it was the practice to operate in three stages, but experience has shown that a colostomy performed for complications can be closed at the same time as the myotomy is performed. Besides sparing patients a third operation, this technique has the theoretical advantage of ensuring that the myotomy is dilated as early as possible by the passage of faeces. This prevents the cut edges of the defunctioned myotomy adhering to one another and ensures that the colonic lumen remains widened.

There have been four deaths in this series; one patient died postoperatively from coronary thrombosis, one from a pulmonary embolus, one from renal failure and one from faecal peritonitis. Hence, only one death is directly attributable to the operation of sigmoid myotomy. This patient developed peritonitis on the fourth day after operation, an emergency defunctioning colostomy was fashioned, the abdomen contained faeces but, despite intensive supportive measures, the patient died. Autopsy revealed that the myotomy was not the cause of the peritonitis but that a diverticulum between the layers of the mesocolon had perforated. It may well be that this diverticulum had been opened inadvertently when the colon was mobilized and that this accident had not been noticed. Hence, the standard operation of resection of the sigmoid would have prevented this death and it must be emphasized that mobilization of the colon must be performed with care if this complication is to be avoided.

The results of these operations have been assessed on clinical grounds alone. The patients have been followed by personal interview and asked about their general health and bowel habit. Their colons have been examined radiologically and by sigmoidoscopy post-operatively. No facilities exist locally for the recording of the intracolonic pressure patterns. Clinically, the benefits of sigmoid myotomy are dramatic. Patients are delighted to pass one or two well formed stools every day and sigmoidoscopy shows that the recto-sigmoid junction is so wide that the instrument can be passed very easily. Occasionally, the lax bowel allows the widely open orifice of a diverticulum to be seen.

Barium enemata show the absence of 'spasm' but, otherwise, the widened colon appears normal. Haustra are present probably because the crescentic folds of muscle are not divided. The diverticula remain but are shorter and have wider necks; changes that go with a lowering of the intracolonic pressures (Painter, 1964).

Reilly believes that diverticular disease is a reversible process early in its development if treated medically with a sane diet. Surgery is called for when this functional and reversible obstruction has become organic and hence irreversible. It is for this reason that the use of sigmoid myotomy has been arbitrarily confined, with rare exceptions, to patients over 50 years of age.

The main indication for myotomy is uncomplicated diverticular disease with long-standing symptoms that make the patients' life a misery. These patients have hitherto been denied surgery because of the risks attendant on resection and on the assumption that their complaints were not sufficiently severe to warrant the risk of major surgery. The results so far show that myotomy provides satisfactory results and carries only a slight risk.

In only four cases has myotomy been unsuccessful; one was the fistula already described and the other three failures were caused by not carrying the myotomy low enough to relieve the obstruction at the recto-sigmoid region. The role of myotomy in the treatment of complicated diverticulitis is not clear. At the present, it seems that myotomy should be reserved for quiescent forms of the disease after adequate medical treatment has been tried. The operation should not be performed in the presence of peritonitis, pus or intestinal obstruction.

THE INDICATIONS FOR SIGMOID MYOTOMY

Reilly (1969) maintains that myotomy is less hazardous and less severe than resection, especially in the old and obese, an opinion supported by those who practise the operation. He emphasizes that myotomy should not be used in acute infective diverticulitis and suggested that myotomy may be useful in the following circumstances:

(1) Troublesome symptoms of longstanding in diverticular disease that have not been relieved by a high-residue diet;

(2) Sigmoid colons that have been inflamed, but have resolved following proximal colostomy, may be saved by myotomy;

(3) When local resection is necessary for fistula, etc., a wide resection may be avoided by coupling limited resection with myotomy above or below the anastomosis. This avoids wide mobilization of the colon and tension on the anastomosis;

(4) When the thickening of the muscle coat extends from the recto-sigmoid right up into the descending colon, a long myotomy incision is easier than a left hemicolectomy.

He stresses that morphine should not be used postoperatively because it raises the intra-colonic pressures and increases the risk of perforation.

Another indication for myotomy was suggested by Daniel and Singh (1969). They used myotomy in conjunction with uretero-colic anastomosis to lower the intracolonic pressures so as to lessen the likelihood of reflux up the transplanted ureters.

Daniel (1969) reported that myotomy was easier to perform if the colon was distended by CO_2 introduced through a rectal tube from a cylinder fitted with a suitable reducing valve. Any minute perforation of the mucosa was detected easily by the sound of escaping gas. Smith, Giannakos and Clarke (1971) found that distension of the proximal colon complicated the post-operative progress of some patients and so they decompressed the large bowel with a tube passed up to the hepatic flexure through a caecostomy. The caecostomy closed spontaneously once normal bowel function had been regained.

THE LATE RESULTS OF COLOMYOTOMY

The immediate results are good. Patients defaecate easily and their symptoms are relieved. Theoretically, the cut edges of the muscle could be drawn together by the contraction of scar tissue so that the effect of the operation would be reduced. Daniel (1969) sutured free grafts of peritoneum to cover the raw area made by the incision in the hope of preventing this later complication, but has not yet reported the long-term effect of this procedure.

Resection of the sigmoid for diverticular disease abolishes symptoms in only 59% of patients (Bolt and Hughes, 1966). The five-year results of myotomy compare favourably with this. Daniel (1969) reported that 96% of 80 patients who had undergone myotomy were symptom-free; 50 of these had been operated on by Reilly and the other 30 constituted his own series. It is possible that this excellent result was partly due to the practice of both Daniels and Reilly of prescribing a high residue diet post-operatively. By contrast, the patients studied by Bolt and Hughes were left on their customary fibre-deficient diet which may account for the persistence of their symptoms after resection.

THE EFFECT OF MYOTOMY ON THE
INTRACOLONIC PRESSURES

(a) The Initial Effect

The effects of myotomy on the intracolonic pressures have been studied at Edinburgh. Attisha and Smith (1969) recorded the intrasigmoid pressures in nine normal patients, 29 with diverticulosis and 14 patients who had been treated by myotomy from one to six months previously. The basal activity in the three groups was similar, confirming the findings of Painter and Truelove (1964a). Feeding caused the diseased sigmoid to react three times as much as the normal and prostigmine evoked high pressures from those segments that bore diverticula (Fig. 62).

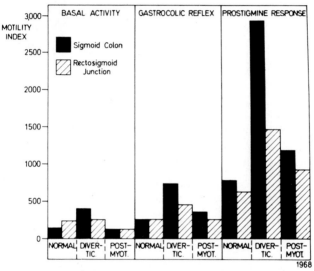

Fig. 62. Response of sigmoid colon in normal patients and in those with diverticular disease and in those who have undergone myotomy. Mean motility indices depicted for basal activity, gastrocolic reflex and prostigmine responses. Motility index = mean wave amplitude × % duration of wave activity, which is a measure of the total pressure produced by the colon. (From Smith, Attisha & Clarke (1971); reproduced by permission of the Editor of the American Journal of Digestive Diseases.)

Myotomy reduced the response to food and more than halved the amount of pressure generated by prostigmine. Analysis showed that myotomy was especially effective in lessening the high waves of pressure in excess of 50 cm./H_2O that are common after prostigmine (Fig. 63).

(b) The Long-Term Effect

Unfortunately, the initial reduction of the intracolonic pressures brought about by myotomy is not permanent. Smith, Attisha and Clarke (1971) followed their patients and recorded

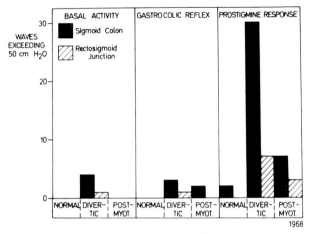

FIG. 63. Number of waves above 50 cm. H₂O pressure. Response of sigmoid colon in normal patients, in patients with diverticular disease and in those who have undergone myotomy. (From Smith, Attisha & Clarke (1971); reproduced by permission of the Editor of the American Journal of Digestive Diseases).

the pressure patterns in their colons at intervals. At the end of three years, the 'motility index' (which is a measure of the total pressure produced by and withstood by the colonic wall), had risen to about 75% of its pre-operative value. Fortunately, this undesirable change was accompanied by the return of few symptoms. Nevertheless, it suggests that the beneficial effects of myotomy are not permanent and that if the operation is performed at an early age, the disease may cause trouble later in life (Fig. 64).

By contrast, they found that resection did not lower these pressures for more than a few months and that at the end of a year the descending colon which, following sigmoidectomy, had become the 'new sigmoid', produced more pressure than had the original diseased sigmoid (Fig. 63). This accords with the work of Parks and Connell (1969) who showed that the diseased sigmoid was weaker in that it was less able to withstand a distending force that was a normal colon. While the organically narrowed sigmoid must be resected, sigmoidectomy appears to have no advantage over myotomy, as regards the intracolonic pressures, if performed for 'hypertrophy' or for painful diverticular disease. This is probably because the descending colon which is anastomosed to the rectum also produces abnormal pressures in diverticular disease (Parks and Connell, 1969).

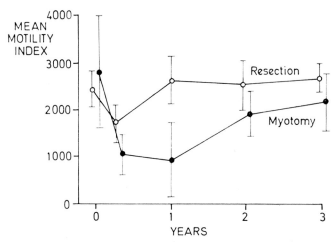

Fig. 64. Mean motility index recorded at 3 months, one, two, and three years of 12 patients treated by resection of the sigmoid and 12 patients treated by sigmoid myotomy. (From Smith, Giannakos & Clarke (1971); by permission of the Editor of the Journal of the Royal College of Surgeons of Edinburgh.)

(c) The Long Term Effect of Myotomy and Resection when accompanied by the taking of a High Fibre Diet

All these patients treated by myotomy or resection, whose motility indices are given in Fig. 63, resumed their normal eating habits after operation. If it is accepted that diverticular disease is caused by a fibre-deficient diet, then these patients who had initially benefited by these procedures were once again subjected to the very stimulus that had caused their disease in the first place. Consequently, it is hardly surprising that after a period of convalescence the colon began to generate high pressures again as it struggled with the small viscous stools that result from an over-refined diet.

In order to see if the removal of this stimulus would benefit patients who had been treated surgically, Smith (1973 and personal communication) persuaded five patients treated by myotomy and 20 patients treated by resection to eat a high-fibre diet including millers' bran after they had left hospital. These patients had the patterns of their intracolonic pressures recorded at intervals post-operatively under similar circumstances, as those who had returned to their former diet, namely at rest, after food and after receiving a dose of prostigmine.

The behaviour of their colons differed markedly after an

operation that was followed by a diet containing a greater amount of fibre. At the end of four years, there was no sign of their intracolonic pressures rising to their former abnormally high levels that they had produced before operation (Figs. 65a and b).

Hence, there is a great contrast between the behaviour of the colons of patients who had continued to consume a fibre-deficient diet and those colons which had to cope with the large soft stools that follow an adequate intake of plant fibre. This being so, surgery, whether it takes the form of myotomy or resection, must be regarded only as an incident, albeit an important one, in the treatment of diverticular disease. The operation should be followed by the taking of an adequate amount of fibre, particularly cereal fibre, so that the patient's colon is not subjected to the diet that caused it to become diseased. This attitude to treatment is comparable to that of a urologist who has treated a bladder neoplasm in an aniline dye worker. He would do his utmost to persuade his patient to change his job so as to avoid this dangerous chemical and so the surgeon who has dealt with diverticular disease should endeavour to improve the environment of his patient's colon by altering his diet. It is my belief that our failure to appreciate this fact has been responsible for the return of symptoms after sigmoidectomy and sigmoid myotomy.

(d) The Place of Motility Studies in the Selection of Patients for Myotomy

The colon that has become rigid due to fibrosis caused by recurrent episodes of diverticulitis is unable to contract and remains open like a drain after the administration of morphine. The muscle surrounding the necks of diverticula arising from such a colon is incapable of contracting so that the colonic contents flow in and out of these diverticula without let or hindrance. This has been demonstrated by cineradiography and pressure studies showed that the scarred sigmoid colon is incapable of producing excessive pressures even when activated by drugs (Painter, 1962). Smith, Attisha and Clarke (1971) confirmed this finding and also noticed that sigmoid colons which had been damaged to this extent did not generate high pressures in response to feeding. They considered that myotomy would be unlikely to be of benefit in these circumstances and that these

RESECTION

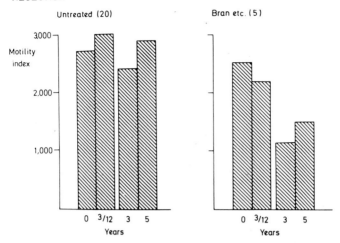

FIG. 65a. The effect of resection coupled with the bran diet. The effect of the taking of food on the motility index of the sigmoid colon was measured before operation (O). After resection of the sigmoid for diverticular disease, the motility index was measured after food at three months, three years and five years; these indices relate to that part of the bowel which has become the 'new' sigmoid. Twenty patients consumed their customary low-fibre diet after resection and it will be seen that the amount of pressure produced by their colons did not alter significantly after resection. By contrast, five patients took a high-fibre diet with bran post-operatively and measurements taken under the same conditions at three and five years showed that the pressure generated by these colons was nearly halved. The significance of these findings is discussed in the text.

rigid colons would be better treated by resection. They therefore suggested that the suitability of patients for myotomy might be determined by the study of their intracolonic pressures before proceeding to operation. Their proposal is logical and deserves further consideration.

TRANSVERSE TAENIO-MYOTOMY

It has been known for at least 70 years that the taeniae are shortened and contracted in diverticular disease with the result that the circular muscle is thrown into folds resembling a concertina, to use Sir Arthur Keith's apt phrase. The colonic lumen is narrowed as a result.

Johnson (1971) founded his operation of 'taenio-myotomy' on this concept. Using New Zealand white rats he cut the taenia coli at regular intervals so as to allow the colon to lengthen,

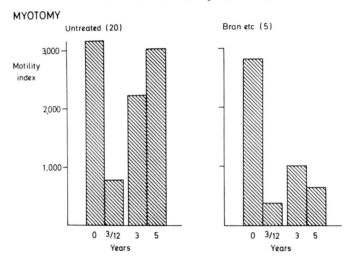

FIG. 65b. The effect of myotomy coupled with the bran diet. The motility index of the sigmoid colon after taking food was measured before and after myotomy at intervals of three months, three and five years. In twenty patients who returned to their customary low-fibre diet, myotomy reduced the postprandial intracolonic pressures but these had returned almost to their former abnormal levels at the end of three years. Five patients were placed on the 'bran diet' after myotomy and, at the end of five years, the beneficial reduction of pressure that followed myotomy was maintained. The significance of these findings is discussed in the text.

become fusiform and so dilated that the haustra could hardly be distinguished. He recorded the intracolonic pressures of these rabbits with water-filled tubes and found that section of the taenia lessened the frequency of the colonic contractions so that its total pressure producing activity was reduced. Hodgson (1973) has applied his work to human subjects by dividing the two antimesocolic taenia at intervals, beginning at the recto-sigmoid junction and proceeding upwards to above the thick-ened part of the sigmoid. He claimed, with some justification, that this form of myotomy was safer as the circular muscle was not divided and so the risk of perforation of the mucosa was minimized, and that the cut edges of the taenia retracted and were less likely to rejoin due to the contraction of scar tissue.The operation has been carried out on 18 patients with two deaths from incidental causes (Hodgson, 1974). As yet, no serious assessment of the results of transverse taenio myotomy has been made and whether this procedure will prove to be useful remains to be seen.

Chapter 21

The Treatment of Diverticular Disease
of the Colon with a High-Fibre Diet

A study of the epidemiology and the historical emergence of
diverticular disease shows that it appears in communities who
have abandoned their traditional eating habits and who have
consumed a diet rich in refined carbohydrates for about 40
years. Food processing, the refining of sugar from beet and the
milling of white flour all result in the removal of plant fibre
from our modern diet. This fibre fraction of our food has been
largely ignored by nutritionists probably because it is 'indigestible' and is of negligible nutrient value. However, it is this fibre
which is least changed by digestion and which reaches the colon
and so influences the environment and the behaviour of the
colon profoundly. A deficiency of dietary fibre alters the consistency of the faecal stream and leads to small hard stools. This
causes the sigmoid colon to segment excessively in order to
generate high pressures in order to propel viscous faeces and
these abnormally high pressures lead to the development of
diverticulosis. By contrast, the addition of cereal fibre, in the
form of unprocessed millers' bran, to the diet results in the
passage of bulky soft stools which can be voided without effort
(Painter, 1964; Painter and Burkitt, 1971; Burkitt, Walker and
Painter, 1972 and 1974).

Thus, diverticulosis coli is caused by the low-residue diet that
has been recommended for its treatment for nearly 50 years,
despite the lack of any convincing evidence that this diet is of
any benefit. In order to see whether the replacement of the
cereal fibre that is missing from our modern over-refined food
would alleviate the symptoms of the disease, Painter, Almeida
and Colebourne (1972) give a high-fibre diet, including unprocessed millers' bran, to 70 patients with symptomatic
diverticular disease. It is important to stress that radiological
examinations had shown that no structural change had caused
stenosis of the colon in any of these patients.

THE REASON FOR PRESCRIBING MILLERS' BRAN

Ideally, a high-fibre diet, or more correctly an unrefined or 'full-fibre' diet, should include plenty of fresh fruit, vegetables and, most important of all, wholemeal bread and flour. Our ancestors who did not get diverticulosis ate this bread in quantity and consumed much less refined sugar (Fig. 66). In the last

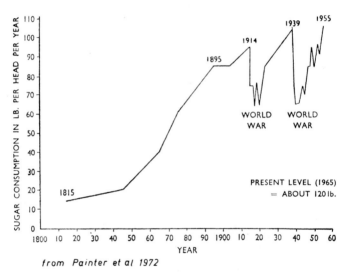

from *Painter et al 1972*

FIG. 66. Rise in sugar consumption in the United Kingdom from 1815 to 1955 (from Cleave, Campbell and Painter, 1969; reprinted by permission of the publisher). The consumption of refined sugar has now risen to about 140 lb. per person annually, that is 6 oz. daily.

hundred years, the total fibre content of the British diet has hardly changed as far as can be ascertained by the information that is available, but its cereal content has dropped by about 2 grams a day according to Robertson (1972). Others, including Trowell (1974 and personal communication) calculate that our intake of cereal fibre has fallen more than this, due to a combination of more efficient milling and to a decrease in the consumption of bread and flour, which began about 1870 and has continued to the present day.

Wheat bran is known to have a laxative effect related to the amount ingested (Cowgill and Anderson, 1932) and its laxative effect exceeds that of fibre derived from fruit and vegetables

(Dimock, 1936). Historically, before the widespread use of canning and the advent of refrigeration, Western man could store only grain products, beans and potatoes for consumption in the winter months, while fruit and most vegetables were eaten only in season. Consequently, it is reasonable to suppose that man's intestinal tract has become adapted to a diet containing cereals almost since the dawn of history and hence it requires a minimum amount of cereal fibre if it is to function properly and to remain healthy.

Unfortunately, it is difficult to obtain an unrefined diet in our modern society. Most people's diet depends on the availability of food at a price that they can afford. This is particularly so in the case of retired people on a fixed income who often can only afford the cheapest foods which are usually those that have been refined and processed to facilitate their transport and storage. Thus, it is fortunate that fibre can be added to the diet cheaply and safely by eating unprocessed millers' bran.

Bran constitutes about 14·5% of the wheat kernel and contains 12·25% fibre, which is about five times that of whole wheat. The safety of All-Bran in the treatment of constipation has long been known and its value has been demonstrated by many, including Dimock (1936) who used it successfully to treat constipation, mucous colitis and spastic colon. Cleave (1941) and personal communication (1967) used millers' bran to relieve constipation, both ashore and afloat, when serving as a consultant physician in the Royal Navy. In 30 years experience, he met no complications due to the taking of bran. In the last eight years bran has been shown to be safe in the treatment of uncomplicated diverticular disease on both sides of the Atlantic and in Italy.

THE EFFECT OF THE 'BRAN DIET' ON SEVENTY PATIENTS

Painter, Almeida and Colebourne (1972) treated 70 unselected patients with diverticular disease with a high-fibre/low sugar diet, together with millers' bran. The trial was not controlled as it would have been unethical for them to prescribe a low-residue diet as they believed that it was the cause of the disease. For practical purposes, the patients acted as their own controls. The trial began at Manor House Hospital in 1967 and was completed by the middle of 1971. Since that time, many more patients have been given bran for diverticulosis with similar results, namely, the relief or abolition of symptoms in nearly 90% of cases. The following paragraphs describe the method of prescribing bran, the instructions given to patients, the effect of the 'bran diet' on bowel behaviour and on the symptoms that bothered these 70 patients.

(a) THE INSTRUCTIONS GIVEN TO PATIENTS

Patients whose symptoms suggest the presence of diverticular or other disease should be investigated accordingly but as soon as diverticula has been demonstrated, the patient should be told of their presence. The nature of their disorder must be explained to them with the aid of a simple diagram (Fig. 67) and its relationship to diet and 'roughage' described briefly. In this way, the patient's confidence is gained and his intelligent co-operation is assured. Some doctors do not tell patients of the presence of diverticula that are causing no symptoms. I believe that this attitude is wrong. Patients are more worried over the unknown and, when they realize that the mucosal 'blowouts' are the result of their diet, they co-operate willingly. As diverticulosis is a progressive disease, symptomatic diverticula should be treated in the hope of preventing complications in the future. Once patients understand that their condition is a benign one that can be treated by simple dietary measures, they are placed on what, for the sake of brevity, is called the 'Bran Diet'.

Each patient is given a packet of unprocessed millers' bran from the hospital dispensary together with a sheet of instructions. This reiterates what they have been told and explains that as bran is difficult to swallow dry, it should be washed down with water, milk or fruit juice or sprinkled on breakfast cereals or mixed with porridge or soup. Bran may also be added to wholemeal flour, in the ratio of one part in five, by those who bake their own bread; the 'bran-plus' loaf that results is very palatable. Patients are advised to eat All-Bran, Weetabix, Shredded Wheat, porridge, fruit and vegetables, especially cabbage. In particular, they are asked to eat 100% wholemeal bread and the difference between this and brown bread is explained to them.

They are asked to reduce their intake of refined sugar, whether brown or white, as this contains no fibre. If patients

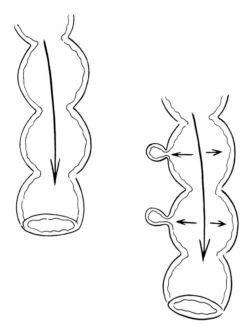

Fig. 67. Simple diagram used to explain bowel physiology to patients. These simple diagrams can be sketched rapidly while explaining to patients how the high residue diet works. The left hand diagram is used for constipation and the right hand diagram to explain the nature of diverticulosis.

With the aid of these diagrams, patients are told that their bowel is a muscular tube which has to segment to produce the pressures which propel faeces through the gut. It is not difficult to make the patients see that if faeces are soft 'like tooth-paste' with a low viscosity they will pass easily through the bowel which will have to exert little effort to propel them. Patients can understand that, by contrast, the small stiff stools of Western man can be propelled through the colon only if considerable force is exerted and that it is the abnormally high pressures involved in this process that cause the mucosa to be forced through the muscle coat rather like 'blow-outs' on a tyre.

Once patients realize that the cramp-like pains and colic which they are ex-periencing are caused by the contraction of the colonic muscle as it struggles with a low-residue diet, they readily understand how a diet that softens their stools will help them. They readily grasp the fact that if they do not have to strain to void soft stools these stools will have passed through the large bowel easily.

Each patient is also told that diverticular disease and constipation is not seen in rural Africans and Asians who eat plenty of fibre and that the object of adding bran to the diet is to replace the fibre that is missing from our modern food.

stop adding sugar to their tea, coffee and other drinks, their consumption of sugar will be significantly reduced. One hundred years ago, when diverticulosis was not a problem, less than half the amount of sugar was eaten than is the case today and, although no direct connection has been demonstrated between sugar and the disease, it seems common sense to limit the intake of a substance that does not appear in nature in its purified state. Women willingly eat less sugar when it is pointed out to them that it merely produces energy, calories or fat!

Patients are then asked to take two teaspoons of millers' bran three times a day and are told that after two weeks they must increase this amount until they open their bowels once or twice a day *without straining*. (If they do not have to strain to defaecate, it is fair to assume that their sigmoid has not had to segment excessively to propel its contents). The amount of bran required to produce this effect must be found by each patient by trial and error. Some patients will need several tablespoonsful of bran each day.

It is essential to warn patients that they may suffer from flatulence when they first take bran.

This will pass off in two or three weeks if they persist with a high-fibre diet, but patients who initially complain of distension may be made temporarily worse by bran and will stop taking it if they are not aware of this transient side effect.

(b) PATIENTS WHO FAIL TO TOLERATE BRAN

Of the 70 patients treated by Painter and his colleagues (1972) three were so improved by changing to wholemeal bread and All-Bran that they did not need bran. This left five who must be classed as failures. Three were nauseated by bran; one was made comfortable with Sterculia (Normacol in this country; Movicol in the United States) and another two sought advice elsewhere. The seventh preferred Normacol to bran and the eighth 'failure' who had taken senna for over 15 years, came to surgery and it was found that his myenteric plexus had been destroyed. Thus, only five failed to benefit from an increased intake of dietary fibre and one of them had a permanently damaged colon. Some patients do not like bran because it gets underneath their dentures. These should take it in soup or porridge so that it is soft and moist when eaten.

(c) THE AMOUNT OF MILLERS' BRAN REQUIRED

The amount of bran required to stop straining at stool varies greatly. This is probably because the amount of fibre in the rest of each patient's diet, and hence its degree of fibre depletion, varies considerably. The dose of bran may vary from one dessertspoon (3 g.) to three tablespoons thrice daily (45 g.). This very high dose is exceptional and on average two teaspoons three times a day (about 12 to 14 g.) of bran renders the stools soft and easy to pass.

Of the 62 patients who took bran, no fewer than 39 (63%) felt distended and suffered from flatulence when they first took bran. This usually disappeared in three weeks but occasionally lasted for eight weeks. In three patients, a sensation of slight distension persisted but they preferred this to their previous symptoms.

(d) THE EFFECT OF THE 'BRAN DIET' ON THE BOWEL HABIT AND CONSISTENCY OF THE STOOLS

The bowel habit of 62 patients with uncomplicated diverticular disease before and after taking the bran diet is shown in Fig. 68. Not only do constipated patients pass soft motions regularly, but those who pass frequent small stools and have attacks of diarrhoea have fewer but soft-formed motions. The Bran Diet not only changes the bowel habit but also alters the consistency of the stools. Before bran, 45 patients out of 62 strained at stool, nine did so sometimes and only eight defaecated without effort. After bran, 51 of the 62 said straining was a thing of the past and only 11 had to exert themselves when emptying their bowels. Sixty said that their stools were softer and two who previously had bouts of diarrhoea reported that their motions had become formed and soft.

A most gratifying effect of bran is that patients frequently say that it enables them to empty their rectum completely whereas formerly they had always felt 'that something was there'. They no longer worry about their bowels and become relaxed. This change in their mental attitude was noticed also by Dimock (1936).

(e) THE REPLACEMENT OF LAXATIVES BY THE BRAN DIET

No less than 49 of the 70 patients with diverticulosis took laxatives when they were first seen; 27 bought them at their own

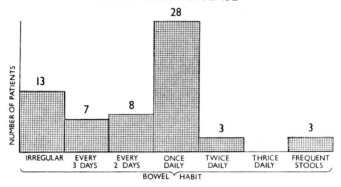

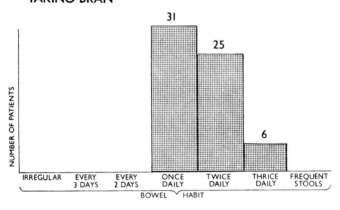

FIG. 68. The effect of a high-fibre diet on the bowel habit in sixty-two patients with diverticular disease (from Painter, Almeida and Colebourne, 1972).

expense and 22 obtained them from their doctor. Of the 62 who took the bran diet only seven needed laxatives and then only occasionally.

A change to bran in the treatment not only of diverticulosis but also of constipation and first-degree haemorrhoids would lead to a great saving of the taxpayers' money. In particular, pensioners on a small income would not squander their meagre resources on expensive medicines if they were to take bran. Furthermore, the long-term abuse of laxatives is not without risks.

(f) DIETARY CHANGES MADE BY INFORMED PATIENTS

Most patients are willing to alter their diet besides taking millers' bran once the reason had been explained to them. They are only too happy to treat their bowels by diet once they understand the reason for it. In our series, 49 changed to whole-meal bread and ate fibre-containing cereals and 14 took porridge regularly.

The bran diet did not change the appetite of 35 patients whose appetite was good, but improved it in 26 whose appetite was poor. The appetite of one, who had previously been treated by a partial gastrectomy, was poor and it remained poor after bran. Not one of our 62 patients was made worse by bran. This surely refutes the widely held view, expressed by no less a person than the late Lord Dawson of Penn and copied without thought by so many authors, that 'roughage' irritates the gut. The fact is that bran when moist becomes 'softage', and this can be confirmed by any doctor who is prepared to try the experiment and take bran himself for a month.

(g) THE RELIEF OF SYMPTOMS BY THE 'BRAN DIET'

Patients with diverticular disease may complain of more than one symptom. Hence, the 70 patients presented with no less than 171 main symptoms. These symptoms may be classified into three groups as has been done in Table 18, they vary from vague 'upper abdominal' symptoms to complaints referring to the rectum. The eight patients who did not take bran experienced 14 (8·2%) of these symptoms. Of the remaining 157 presenting symptoms only six (3·8%) were not relieved by bran and were treated with Normacol. Sixty-two (39·5%) symptoms were relieved and the remaining 89 (56·7%) symptoms disappeared once it had taken effect. A similar result was obtained by Plumley and Francis (1973) who gave their patients about 13 g. of bran daily in the form of a high-fibre biscuit.

Thus a simple change of diet relieved or abolished the symptoms of uncomplicated diverticular disease in 88·6% of the patients.

Bran will cure not only constipation but also diarrhoea. Frequent small motions or episodes of diarrhoea, sometimes the result of using laxatives, were the main problem of seven patients. All were improved. One who defaecated 12 times a day and another who did so six times a day passed motions but twice a day on the bran diet. A further patient who passed three soft motions a day on bran preferred this to episodic diarrhoea and the abdominal discomfort of which he had complained previously.

(h) THE EFFECT OF THE BRAN DIET ON PAINFUL AND COMPLICATED DIVERTICULAR DISEASE

Two patients had 'acute diverticulitis' before taking bran, but as they both had a normal white count they should have been classified as having 'painful diverticular disease' (Painter, 1968). A third had attacks of 'left renal colic' which proved to be of colonic origin. All three have remained well since they have taken a high-fibre diet. It must be emphasized that this regimen does not prevent attacks of painful diverticular disease or acute diverticulitis. Three of the 62 patients whose symptoms had been relieved and were established on the high-fibre diet were admitted to hospital with pain and tenderness in the left iliac fossa. Only one had acute suppurative diverticulitis and all recovered with conservative treatment. As soon as the emergency was over and they were allowed to eat, they were given bran and have remained on it since; the state of their colon was re-assessed by barium enema when the tenderness had disappeared.

Twelve patients had recurrent attacks of painful diverticular disease characterized by severe colic and that made them potential candidates for surgery (Table 18). One would not take bran but was made comfortable with Normacol, while, in four the colic was relieved and in seven it was abolished by the bran diet. Despite having severe pain formerly, none have come to surgery, although there is no doubt that a few years ago some of them would have been treated by sigmoid resection in the mistaken belief that they had 'diverticulitis'. One of the 12 was a lady of 50 who had been given pethidine (demerol) on three occasions for left renal colic. Repeated examinations showed her urinary tract to be normal and a barium enema revealed a very active sigmoid beset with diverticula. She was then placed on a high-fibre diet and has not suffered from severe pain for over five years. It is unlikely that this is because she has not passed another small stone because she experiences mild cramp in the left iliac fossa occasionally which is in the same position as her former severe colic and it varies in its

TABLE 18

		Before Bran	Bran Not Tolerated	Symptoms after Bran Not Relieved	Relieved	Abolished
Dyspeptic Symptoms	Nausea	11	1	1	2	7
	Heartburn	2	—	—	2	—
	Flatulence	2	—	1	1	—
	Distension	36	4	2	14	16
	Wind	13	—	—	4	9
Painful Diverticular Disease	R.I.F. pain or ache	7	—	0	5	2
	L.I.F. pain or ache	22	1	1	7	13
	Lower or general abdominal pain	28	3	—	11	14
	Severe colic	12	1	—	4	7
Bowel symptoms	Tender rectum	4	—	—	1	3
	Incomplete emptying of rectum	6	—	—	3	3
	Constipation	28	4	1	8	15
	Total symptoms	171	14	6	62	89

The presenting symptoms of seventy patients with diverticular disease. The seventy patients complained of 171 main symptoms. Fourteen belonged to patients who did not take bran. Only 6 (3·8%) of symptoms were not relieved by bran.

intensity with the same periodicity as did the severe colic. This disappears if she doubles her intake of bran for a few days.

Thus, even severe colic that formerly would have led to surgery will respond to a high-fibre diet. Moreover, this treatment is both cheaper and safer than the long-term use of conventional laxatives which is not without risk. Paraffin and hydrophylic colloids have disadvantages, and the prolonged use of senna destroys the colon's intrinsic nerve supply (Smith, 1968). The widespread use of bran would lessen the need for surgery in diverticular disease.

The Origin of the Symptoms of Diverticular Disease

The beneficial effects of bran on the symptoms of diverticular disease are not only of practical importance but are also of theoretical interest. The symptoms of diverticular disease can be grouped, in descending order of magnitude, into those associated with

(1) *Acute Diverticulitis*—the symptoms of which vary according to the damage that is wrought by the inflammatory process;

(2) *Painful Diverticular Disease*—the colic of this condition waxes and wanes too rapidly to be due to inflammation and is now attributed to intermittent functional obstruction of the colon brought about by excessive colonic segmentation (Painter, 1964 and 1968);

(3) *Diverticulosis*—vague symptoms such as a sense of fullness, flatulence, abdominal distension and aching, a loss of appetite and alteration in the bowel habit may all be associated with the presence of colonic diverticula.

The symptoms of diverticulosis cannot be due to the presence of diverticula alone as both a high-residue diet and Reilly's operation will relieve symptoms without removing these mucosal herniations. Although severe colic is known to be due to abnormal activity of the colonic muscle, the place of origin of these less specific symptoms is uncertain. Their relief by the bran diet may throw some light on their cause. If a fibre-deficient diet can damage the colon to such an extent that it 'ruptures' itself through struggling with its abnormal contents, is it not extremely unlikely that this is the only part of the intestinal tract to be adversely affected by our modern diet? This over-refined diet is so new in the time-scale of human nutrition that it would be hardly surprising if our gut had not yet adapted to it. Is it not possible, therefore, that some of the symptoms of diverticulosis originate in other parts of the intestine which also have to struggle with an unnatural diet and whose motility is altered by this diet?

This concept, namely that the whole of the alimentary tract has to struggle with a low residue diet, explains not only why 'upper intestinal' symptoms accompany diverticulosis but also how the high-fibre diet relieves symptoms which appear to arise at different levels of the gastro-intestinal tract.

CONCLUSION

The fact that a high-fibre diet alleviates the symptoms of diverticular disease does not prove that the disease is caused by fibre-deficiency. This has been pointed out by those who have a vested interest in defending the white flour and sliced bread that is sold to the public today. It has also been claimed that the fibre content of the British diet has hardly changed in the last hundred years.

This is not the place to debate the differing figures that have been presented by nutritionists, but it is obvious that if the addition of only two to three grams of cereal fibre has such a profound effect on the behaviour of the human intestine, those who believe that fibre-deficiency is important do not have to prove that a great drop in dietary fibre has occurred. It would appear that the human colon had adapted to the partial refining of food over many centuries. but that towards the end of the last century the amount of fibre in the diet dropped below the level necessary for the correct and healthy functioning of our gut. If this is accepted, then we should retrace our dietary footsteps and insist, by legislation if necessary, that our bread must provide us with a few grams of cereal fibre each day.

Chapter 22

Dietary Fibre, Diverticulosis and its Associated Diseases

In many parts of the world, the pattern of disease that is prevalent locally has changed dramatically in the last century. Formerly, the infectious diseases led to a high mortality amongst the young but advances in public health in the industrialized nations of the West, followed 40 years ago by the sulpha drugs and later by the antibiotics, have almost conquered these diseases. The same results of medical progress have been observed in the developing countries in recent years.

Unfortunately, this great achievement is something of a Pyrrhic victory because the same technological discoveries that led to the eradication of the infectious diseases has also altered the pattern of life and the eating habits of those nations which have been its chief beneficiaries. Consequently, their citizens are now prone to several degenerative diseases which include diabetes, atherosclerosis, coronary artery disease, cancer of the colon, diverticular disease, gall-stones and other less serious conditions. The expectancy of life at birth has increased in the Western countries so that a greater proportion of their populations reach middle age but, despite this initial advantage, their life expectancy calculated in the prime of life has altered for the better but little in recent years. By contrast, the South African black who survives to the age of 50 can look forward to more years of active healthy life than can his white compatriots. This is because all these degenerative diseases are extremely rare to this very day in the rural communities of Africa and Asia (Burkitt, 1973; Cleave, Campbell and Painter, 1969; Walker, 1964 and personal communication).

This disappointing and somewhat paradoxical state of affairs is seen only in the industrialized nations of the West where these degenerative diseases have become common in this century. However, there are signs that history is repeating itself because a similar change in the pattern of disease is occurring wherever economic development has interfered with the traditional way of life. Already, these modern diseases of the West are being detected in the urban citizens of Africa and Asia, while they remain almost unknown in rural communities. Historically, a change in the pattern of disease occurred in this country and the U.S.A. in the last century similar to that which is presently becoming manifest in those countries who are imitating our way of life.

All races and ethnic groups appear to be equally vulnerable to these diseases. West Indian immigrants in Britain and the American Negro are as prone to these diseases as are their white compatriots and rural Africans who are of the same stock suffer from them when they adopt a Western way of life. Similarly, they have been almost unknown in Japan until recently although they affect Japanese-Americans who have been reared in Hawaii and in the continental United States very frequently.

These 'modern' degenerative diseases appeared on the clinical scene too suddenly to be attributed to a widespread genetic change in whole populations and so they must be due to factors which have altered the environment to an extent to which the human body has not been able to adapt. While it must always be remembered that 'civilization' has changed the pattern of our lives so that we take less exercise, inhale fumes, smoke cigarettes and are subjected to the stresses linked with urban living, it is still probable that the major factor affecting our environment is the food that we eat.

DIETARY CHANGES OF THIS CENTURY

The calorie intake of our diet has increased in the last century, more total protein is eaten and a greater proportion of it is derived from animals. Fat consumption has increased. The total unrefined carbohydrate content of our diet has decreased because less bread and cereals are eaten and these are now of low extraction. Concurrently, the intake of refined sugar has increased several-fold.

Formerly, the poor subsisted on a diet containing a large amount of bread made from stoneground flour supplemented by a little meat and vegetables, but around the year 1880 improvements in rail and sea transport and in refrigeration resulted in a greater variety of foods being made available even to the poorer classes. The benefits of the industrial revolution caused wages to rise in value, so that foods which previously had been the prerogative of the rich were eaten by the many in preference to the cereal products which had previously been eaten. This was because they were more attractive to the palate or to the eye.

At the same time, a reduction in import duty led to an increase in the consumption of sugar from the West Indies and the newly popular processing of beet made refined sugar one of the cheapest sources of calories. Bread, which had been made of wholemeal flour or 'white' flour from which the bran had been extracted by sifting, altered as the introduction of roller-milling led to even finer flour from which most of the little remaining fibre was removed.

More efficient refining coupled with a decrease in the consumption of bread caused the cereal fibre content of our diet to drop dramatically. Some observers claim that the total plant fibre in our diet has hardly altered in the last century, but even they would admit that the consumption of fruit and vegetables, many of which were formerly available only when in season, has increased. Consequently, it is obvious that the amount of fibre derived from cereals in our diet has been reduced when compared with that which was eaten by our ancestors (Table 19). As it has been shown that the addition of 2 g. of cereal fibre to the diet affects the colon profoundly altering both the frequency of defaecation and the consistency of the stools, it seems likely that our dietary fibre was reduced below a critical level during this time so that the sudden fall in fibre that then took place did not have to be very great to lead to serious consequences (Walker, 1961 and 1974; Barker, McKenzie and Yudkin, 1966; Cleave, Campbell and Painter, 1969; Painter, 1972a and b; Painter, 1973; Painter, Almeida and Colebourne, 1972; Robertson, 1972; Payler, 1973; Trowell—personal communication).

THE EFFECT OF FIBRE ON THE INTESTINAL TRANSIT TIMES AND THE BULK AND VISCOSITY OF THE STOOLS

In those countries where the degenerative diseases are rare, the natural amount of dietary fibre is eaten and results in large

TABLE 19

	1880		*1970*		*Changes in fibre intake*
	Food	Fibre	Food	Fibre	
Starches:					
Cereals	480	3·2[1]	120	0·3	−90%
Potatoes	300	1·1	120	0·5	−45%
Legumes	60	1·0	60	1·0	None
Starchy fibre	—	5·3	—	1·8	−66%
Fruit and vegetables	275	2·8	325	3·3	+20%
Total fibre	—	8·1	—	5·1	−37%

[1] Assumed fibre content of bread 0·7 g. per 100 g. (i.e. about 85% extraction; roller mills had only just started in U.S.A.).
Prepared by Dr. H. C. Trowell from material of Antar *et al.* (1964).
Amer. J. Clin. Nutrition 14: 169.

soft stools that traverse the intestine rapidly. By contrast, the refined low-fibre foods of the economically developed countries produce small firm stools of greater viscosity which pass through the gut slowly. The time taken by food and its residues to pass through the intestine can be measured by timing the passage of millet seeds, carmine or barium salts but these methods have been superseded by that of Hinton *et al.* (1969) which gives reproducible results. Twenty-five radio-opaque plastic pellets, about the size of rice grains, 2–3 mm. in length, are swallowed after a meal and the next five or six stools are voided into numbered plastic bags and the time at which each stool is passed is recorded. The stools are then weighed and x-rayed. The time elapsing between swallowing and passing 20 (80%) of the pellets is calculated and is called the TRANSIT TIME. One or two pellets may stay in the bowel for many days and the passage of 20 pellets gives reliable results. In rural hospitals, where facilities are limited, the pellets can be retrieved by sieving thus avoiding the need for x-rays.

Table 20 shows the daily stool weight and transit times in groups of various races in different countries. The range of values in one group often overlaps the results obtained from another group. This variation is probably due to personal

TABLE 20
TRANSIT-TIMES AS SHOWN BY HINTON'S METHOD

Subjects	Country	Race	Type of diet	No. of subjects	Time of appearance of first pellets (hr.)		Transit-time (hr.)		Weight of stools passed per day (g.)		Comments
					Range	Mean	Range	Mean	Range	Mean	
Naval ratings and wives	U.K.	White	Refined	15	22–110	45·7	44–144	83·4	39–223	104	Shore-based personnel (compare Steigman)
Teenage boarding-school pupils	U.K.	White	Refined	9	18–103	57·4	35–120	76·1	71–142	110	Institutional diet together with cakes, sweets, and so on from school shop
Students	South Africa	White	Refined	100	13–54	30·5	28–60	48·0	120–195	173	These ate more fruit than is usual in the U.K.
Nurses	South Indian	Indian	Mixed	13	9–34	27·6	23–64	44·0	—	155	Less refined diet than that of Western world
Urban school-children	South Africa	African	Mixed	500	9–40	28·5	24–59	45·2	120–260	165	Partly Europeanized diet
Manor House Hospital patients	U.K.	White	Mixed	6	15–24	22·0	27–48	41·0	128–248	175	U.K. diet plus wholemeal bread and added bran
Senior boarding-school pupils	Uganda	African	Mixed	27	4–54	27·6	22–118	47·0	48–348	185	Traditional Ugandan diet plus refined sugar, white bread, jam, butter

Vegetarians	U.K.	White	Mixed	24	8–49	22·0	18–97	42·4	71–488	225	Note similarity of values to those of African groups
Rural school-children	South Africa	African	Un-refined	500	5–28	12·8	20–48	33·5	150–350	275	—
Rural villagers	Uganda	African	Un-refined	15	4–32	19·8	19–68	35·7	178–980	470	Villagers not yet supplementing their diet with processed foods of Western type

physical factors and personal dietary preferences which are indulged within the limits of the foodstuffs available locally.

On average, the more refined the diet the smaller and slower is the pasage of food residues through the intestine. By contrast, diets rich in fibre produce bulky, soft stools which traverse the gut rapidly. The fibre-deficient food residues of Western man may remain in the bowel for several days and yet be associated with a daily bowel movement. Hence, there is truth in the old adage that a patient may be regular but five days late.

There is an inverse relationship between daily stool weights and transit times (Fig. 69). The bulky stool containing more

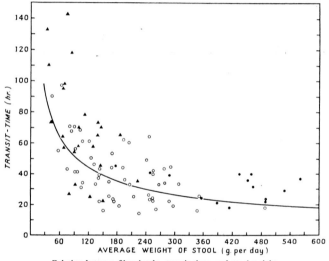

Relation between fibre intake, transit-time, and stool weight.
O = Vegetarians, vegans, and African boarding-school (mixed diet).
● = African villagers (high-residue diet).
▲ = English boarding-school and British Navy (low-residue diet).
The curve (which is based on more data than the points shown here) is:
log (time) = 2·81633−0·56057 log (weight).

Fɪɢ. 69.

fibre weighs more and is propelled through the bowel faster. This is true regardless of race. British vegetarians have stool weights and patterns of bowel behaviour that are essentially similar to Ugandan boarding-school pupils. Both groups may be said to be on a 'mixed' diet, that is a diet not as refined as that of whites in the U.K. or U.S.A. but more refined than that of the Ugandan villager (Burkitt, Walker and Painter, 1972 and

1974). Similar results were obtained in Rhodesia by Holmgren and Mynors (1972).

The addition of bran to the diet of British patients produced stools of about the same weight and similar transit times as had been found in these two groups (Table 20). This effect has been confirmed by Parks (1973) and by Payler (1973) while Harvey, Pomare and Heaton (1973) found that 4 g. of bran fibre daily not only corrected constipation but also increased the transit time if it had previously been short. This supports the findings of Painter and his colleagues (1972) who reported that bran fibre cured both constipation and episodes of diarrhoea in patients with diverticulosis. McCance and Widdowson (1956) and Manoussos and his colleagues (1967) found that transit times were increased by about 24 hours by eating white instead of brown bread.

The addition of dietary fibre in the form of bran has two other important effects. First, it decreases the viscosity of the faeces so that it is no longer necessary for patients to strain at stool which must mean that their colons have not had to segment excessively to propel their contents and, second, patients who take a sufficiency of bran-fibre report that they empty their rectums completely and no longer feel that 'something is always there' throughout the day. This leads not only to physical but also to mental relaxation and rest (Dimock, 1936; Painter, Almeida and Colebourne, 1972; Burkitt, Walker and Painter, 1972).

The increase in the weight of the stools that follows the use of bran is due to its ability to retain water in the bowel. This in turn lessens the viscosity of the faeces and dilutes the faecal bile salts although the total output of bile acids and of fats in the faeces is unaltered (Eastwood *et al.*, 1973; Parks, 1973). There is no evidence that bran leads to calcium deficiency or to a decreased absorption of fat or of protein in the small intestine, (Walker, 1972 and 1974—in the press).

Dietary fibre has been defined as that part of the plant material that is ingested in our diet but which resists digestion by the human gastrointestinal tract and so is voided in the faeces (Trowell, 1972). This is not the same as the 'crude' fibre of the chemists, which is that part of a foodstuff remaining after treatment with boiling acids and alkalis, processes that can be carried out in the laboratory but not in the human body. The role of dietary fibre has been reviewed recently by Cummings (1973).

DIETARY FIBRE AND THE PATTERN OF DISEASE

Disquiet over the appearance of these 'new' diseases was voiced in Britain before the beginning of this century by Brunton, Treves, McEwan and later by Sir Robert McCarrison, whose enthusiasm led to the foundation of the Indian Institute of Nutrition. In the United States, Charles Mayo maintained that alterations which had occurred in the quality of food were responsible for the appearance of appendicitis (Walker, 1974). Inevitably, attempts have been made to connect certain disorders with some fraction of the diet, the relationship between cholesterol and coronary artery disease being but one example. As yet, these attempts have yielded mainly inconclusive results probably because these disorders are not due to a single factor.

Cleave and Yudkin, working independently, assert that the increased consumption of refined sugar is responsible for most 'modern' diseases (Cleave, Campbell and Painter, 1969; Cleave, 1974; Yudkin, 1972) while others argue that too much fat or too much protein in the diet are dangerous (Childs, 1972).

Although its importance has long been recognized in animal husbandry, dietary fibre had been largely ignored by nutritionists until Walker (1961, 1969 and 1974) in South Africa pointed out that a correlation existed between certain diseases and a diet depleted of fibre. Trowell (1960) described the non-infective diseases of the native African and drew attention to differences in the fibre consumption of the African villager, his urban counterpart and the European community. He stressed the extreme rarity of diverticulosis, of piles and of the irritable or spastic colon and put forward the hypothesis that absence of these colonic diseases in Africans might well be due to, 'a soft bulky stool and a placid temperament'. Even Cleave, who regards refined sugar as the arch criminal and who has assigned only a secondary role to dietary fibre, would agree with this because he has advocated the use of millers' bran for treating constipation for over 30 years. He claims to have 'introduced unprocessed bran into human therapeutics' (Cleave, 1973) and it was he who first persuaded the author to use unprocessed bran. From this followed the idea of treating uncomplicated diverticular disease with bran (Painter, 1969).

At the same time, Burkitt (1969 and 1973) began to amass data from hospitals all over the world but, particularly, from

Africa, where he had spent his clinical life, showing that these degenerative diseases of civilization are prevalent wherever a fibre-depleted diet is eaten. These diseases always appear together in a population heralded by appendicitis which affects younger people. These diseases never appear singly in a population but always are found together. Often they affect the same patient. They are rare in rural communities who eat unrefined foods but appear in them when they change their eating habits as a result of socio-economic development. The value of bran in the treatment of constipation and of diverticulosis supports his contention that a 'return to a high-residue diet could have an effect on the health of the Western nations as beneficial as would be the elimination of cigarette smoking'.

Neither Walker, Burkitt, Trowell nor any of those who are interested in fibre, would claim that the addition of a few grams of fibre to our diet would cure all our ills or that a deficiency of dietary fibre is the sole cause of the diseases which are associated with diverticular disease. However, if it is accepted that dietary fibre is connected with the development of colonic diverticula and that it will relieve the symptoms that accompany them, then it must be admitted that fibre may play a role in the causation of those conditions which are always associated with diverticular disease. Already, observations have been made that support this submission. Some of them are given in the next paragraphs.

DISEASES OF CIVILIZATION THAT ARE ASSOCIATED WITH DIVERTICULOSIS

Fibre-deficiency has been shown to alter the mechanics of bowel behaviour. Thus, there is no doubt that it may alter the physiology and the environment of the intestine by lessening the time available for metabolic and bacterial processes to take place within its lumen. A sufficiency of fibre which swells when moist and forms a gel may alter the conditions under which absorption takes place. Thus, fibre affects not only the motility of the gut but also the whole of human metabolism. The direct and indirect effects of fibre-depletion and their possible role in the causation of several diseases that are associated with diverticulosis will now be discussed.

(a) Metabolic Diseases that May be Influenced by Dietary Fibre

(i) OBESITY

Unrefined foods are bulky and fill the stomach, and thus assuage the appetite. Food refining concentrates carbohydrates and allows an excess of calories to be eaten. Furthermore, refined sugar given to children leads to a 'sweet tooth' and this addiction is hard to cure (Cleave, Campbell and Painter, 1969; Cleave, 1974). Heaton (1973) points out that fibre provides three obstacles to excess caloric intake. First, it displaces available nutrients from the diet. Second, fibre makes chewing necessary and this slows down the intake of food, promotes the secretion of saliva and gastric juice, thus distending the stomach and leading to satiety. By contrast, refined sugars can be drunk in solution and do not have this effect. Third, fibre decreases the rate of absorption of nutrients in the small intestine. He believes the refining of food increases its 'energy/satiety' ratio and that this may account for the prevalence of obesity in the Western nations.

(ii) DIABETES MELLITUS

Cleave and Campbell believe that not only can refined carbohydrates be eaten to excess but that sugar in this form is absorbed from the bowel with an abnormal rapidity. This in turn leads to a high blood glucose which places an excessive strain on the pancreas. Observations on the Indian population of Natal show that an excess intake of refined sugar is followed by a rise in the incidence of diabetes within 20 years (Cleave, Campbell and Painter, 1969). The strong association between diabetes, diverticulitis and cardiovascular disease was demonstrated by Schowengerdt and his colleagues (1969) in both black and white Americans. This is consistent with the view that fibre deficiency may play a part in the causation of all these three conditions.

(iii) ATHEROMA, ISCHAEMIC HEART DISEASE AND CHOLELITHIASIS

These conditions have been found to co-exist frequently with diverticular disease (Hughes, 1969; Kyle, 1968; Painter *et al.*, 1972). The association of diverticulosis, hiatus hernia and gallstones is known as Saint's Triad. Diverticulosis and ischaemic heart disease have a similar epidemiology and historically they emerge on the clinical scene together (Trowell, Painter and Burkitt, 1974). Hence, it is possible that the removal of fibre from foodstuffs not only helped to cause diverticulitis, which first appeared in the Registrar General's reports as a cause of death in 1923, but may also be partly responsible for the appearance of coronary artery thrombosis in these reports in 1926 and for the greatly increased incidence of gall-stones containing cholesterol (Burkitt, Walker and Painter, 1972 and 1974).

It has been suggested by Trowell (1972a and b) that a high-fibre intake increases faecal steroid output and that, as this is the main metabolic pathway in man for the excretion of cholesterol, the blood cholesterol is lowered thus lessening the chances of atheroma or gall-stones containing cholesterol developing. Attempts have been made to alter the blood lipids by feeding fibre but so far have proved inconclusive (Eastwood, 1969; Cummings, 1973; Heaton and Pomare, 1974).

(iv) PEPTIC ULCERATION

The increased incidence of duodenal ulceration which has occurred in this century has been attributed to the 'stress of modern life'. This implies that our ancestors suffered little stress or that a sudden genetic change has led to a widespread production of an excessive amount of acid and gastric juice. A moment's reflection will reveal that both propositions are nonsense.

Cleave (1962) points out that 'acid-pepsin aggression versus the mucosal defence' equation has blinded the profession to the buffering properties of protein. He maintains that the refining of carbohydrates strips protein from our food so that an excess of acid remains in the stomach. Some experimental support for this view was provided by Lennard-Jones, Fletcher and Shaw (1968) who found that unrefined grain products caused a steeper climb in gastric acidity than did their unrefined counterparts. Peptic ulcer occurs in communities who eat refined carbohydrates and Cleave has collected data from prison camps in the Far East in 1942–45. In Singapore and Hong Kong, where polished rice was given to prisoners of war, duodenal ulcer became a 'plague'. By contrast, in a camp near Tokyo which was subjected to the stress of heavy aerial bombardment, no case was seen in 6,000 prisoners in one year. Here, unmilled barley and millet formed much of the diet (Cleave, Campbell and Painter, 1969).

Tovey (1971 and 1972) studied duodenal ulceration in the workers on tea estates in Southern India where polished rice is eaten. These ulcers differ from those seen in England in that they affect younger people, are less prone to bleed on to perforate and more frequently lead to fibrosis and pyloric stenosis. He gave pasteurized bran as a supplement to the diet of 45 who suffered from duodenal ulcer and 58% of them were relieved of their symptoms. Considering the fact that many duodenal ulcers have caused chronic scarring and narrowing of the pylorus by the time they are diagnosed, this result is most encouraging. It is well known that wholemeal bread stops in the stomach longer and the author has found that the few 'early' ulcers that are referred to him for a surgical opinion often respond to a high-fibre/low-sugar diet and believes that a trial of an unrefined diet containing only 100% wholemeal bread should be undertaken by physicians who see peptic ulceration in its early stages.

(b) Diseases which are Related to Small Viscous Stools and Prolonged Transit Times

(i) APPENDICITIS

Rendle Short (1920) produced evidence that appendicitis was due to a lack of roughage in the diet. A low residue diet has been shown to produce viscous stools which may well cause excessive pressures to be produced in the appendix. If these are of sufficient magnitude, they would devitalize the mucosa so as to permit the entry of organisms into the tissues. Appendicitis has the same epidemiology as diverticular disease and colonic tumours but, because it is a disease that affects the young, precedes their appearance in populations who adopt Western eating habits by about 20 years (Burkitt, 1971). Walker and his colleagues (1973) found that the incidence of appendicectomy scars in South African teenagers varied. The higher the fibre content of their diet, the less was the frequency of appendicitis. Only 0·5% of rural African students had suffered from appendicitis, 0·9% of peri-urban Africans, 1·4% of urban Africans and 2·9% of the Indian population. By contrast, no less than 16·5% of Caucasian students had appendicectomy scars. They also studied no less than 1,325 Caucasian students living in institutions whose diet contained more fibre but less fat and sugar. They defaecated more often, had shorter transit times than their more fortunate Caucasian counterparts and had only 23% of their incidence of appendicectomy scars. It was concluded that appendicitis was environmental in origin and probably related to dietary fibre.

(ii) BENIGN AND MALIGNANT TUMOURS OF THE COLON

Both polyps and cancer of the colon are common in Europe and in those of European stock who have emigrated to the industrialized and predominantly white countries. American Negroes, West Indians in Britain and Japanese Americans are all as prone to these tumours as are their white compatriots (Table 21). In the Western world, cancer of the colon is second only to cancer of the lung as a killing neoplasm. These tumours have the same epidemiology as does diverticular disease and are almost unknown in primitive communities to this day (Burkitt, 1971, 1973a and b; Painter and Burkitt, 1971; Stemmerman and Yatani, 1973).

Fibre may play a part in the causation of these tumours because it has been shown that the faecal bacteria of Americans

TABLE 21

AGE-STANDARDIZED INCIDENCE RATES FOR CANCER OF THE COLON AND RECTUM IN MEN 35–64 YEARS OF AGE ARRANGED IN ORDER OF INCIDENCE (MODIFIED FROM DOLL, 1969). THE VARIATIONS IN THE RATIO OF RECTAL/COLON TUMOURS ARE SHOWN BY THE BLACK DOTS ON THE SAME SCALE. 100 = PARITY.

(From Burkitt, 1973)

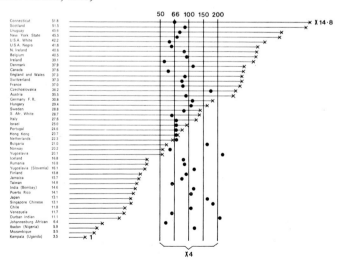

and Britons degrade bile to form the precursors of carcinogens. This does not apply to the faecal flora of Ugandans, Indians and Japanese (Aries *et al.*, 1969; Hill *et al.*, 1971). The role of bacteria and bile degradation has still to be evaluated, but it is reasonable to suggest that the high-fibre diet of the Ugandan, who does not suffer from colonic neoplasms, would speed the elimination of the faeces and dilute them so that any noxious chemicals would remain in contact with the colonic mucosa for less time and in a lower concentration when compared with that of Westerners. Hence, there are at least good theoretical grounds for taking a diet rich in fibre (Burkitt, Walker and Painter, 1972 and 1974; Walker and Walker, 1969). The addition of bran to the diet will reduce the degradation of bile salts (Pomare and Heaton, 1973) and using labelled bile salts, Heaton (personal communication) has shown that bran will reduce their degradation in British patients to the level that is found in Nigerians in whom colonic neoplasms are rare. Falaiye (1974) has confirmed that Nigerians produce less desoxycholate than Europeans. These observations all accord with the proposition that a high-fibre diet lessens the chances of the colon and its mucosa undergoing neoplastic change.

(iii) THE 'IRRITATED' BOWEL SYNDROME

One of the commonest syndromes is that of abdominal pain accompanied by constipation or diarrhoea and sometimes the passage of mucus per rectum. No organic abnormality can be demonstrated in the bowel and symptoms are attributed to an 'irritable' or 'spastic' colon. However, there is no proof that these symptoms are of only colonic origin and so the term 'irritable bowel syndrome' has gained acceptance because the function of the small intestine as well as the large bowel is disturbed and produces waves of high pressure (Holdstock, Misiewicz and Walker, 1969). This symptom-complex is so ill-defined that one wonders if it is really an entity. All agree that the function of the intestine is disturbed but no structural abnormality has been demonstrated to account for the genuine symptoms that are attributed to the irritable gut.

As no evidence of any intrinsic abnormality in the intestine has been found, could it not be that the bowel is normal and the symptoms are caused by its having to struggle with an abnormal diet which is fibre-deficient? In my experience over six years, a high-fibre/low-sugar diet relieves the symptoms of the condition in over 80 % of patients in whom no diverticula or other abnormality have been demonstrated. Recently, Piepmeyer (1974) has relieved the pain of the irritable bowel syndrome in 23 out of 30 patients by adding bran to the diet. It is of interest that the syndrome is almost unknown in rural Africa where an unrefined diet is eaten (Trowell, 1960).

The term 'irritable' bowel syndrome implies that the design or the construction of the intestine is faulty and that it cannot cope with the stresses of everyday life. It seems very unlikely that this can be so as over half the patients who attend gastro-intestinal clinics are said to suffer from this condition. It seems far more likely that, owing to evolution and natural selection, the bowel is normal and the symptoms are caused by our over-refined low-residue diet. Hence, it would be wiser to use the term *'irritated'* bowel syndrome (Painter, 1972). This would shift attention away from what is probably a normal bowel towards the sensible eating habits that would relieve the symptoms of these 'unruly guts' (Godding, 1972). It is the author's practice to prescribe a high-fibre diet to patients with the 'irritated bowel syndrome'.

(c) Some other Conditions which are associated with a Low Fibre Diet

These diseases are not connected with the alimentary tract but may be related indirectly to the alterations in intestinal behaviour that follow the ingestion of a low fibre diet. The stools resulting from such a diet are small and viscous and frequently they are voided only with an effort, which raises the intra-abdominal pressure sometimes to 200 mg/Hg or more.

(i) VARICOSE VEINS

The idea that these are due to man's erect posture, to an hereditary factor or to pregnancy is completely incompatible with the epidemiology of varicose veins (Burkitt, 1972, 1973; Cleave, Campbell and Painter, 1969). Varicose veins and deep vein thrombosis occur in countries who eat refined foods and are rare where a full-fibre diet is still eaten.

Cleave maintains that, in constipated people, the loaded colon presses on the pelvic veins so as to hinder the return of blood from the legs. This relationship may hold good in dissecting room cadavers but the author is certain that it does not do so in life, having palpated the colon at operation to check the truth or otherwise of this belief. It is more likely that repeated straining at stool raises the intra-abdominal pressure to an abnormal extent and that this pressure, being transmitted to the leg veins, damages their valves. The subsequent development of varices is then inevitable (Burkitt, 1972).

The prevalence of varicose veins is significantly greater in patients with diverticular disease, which supports the view that the two conditions have causative factors in common (Latto, Wilkinson and Gilmore, 1973).

(ii) HAEMORRHOIDS

These are related epidemiologically to constipation and varicose veins. Straining at stool would favour the prolapse of veins in the anal canal and hinder their emptying. Moreover, hard balls of faeces would exert local pressure on the submucosal rectal veins causing them to become distended. It is the author's practice to give bran before and after haemorrhoidectomy. First, and some second-degree piles will become symptom-free once their proud owner is established on an adequate dose of bran. This saves operating and supports the view that an easily passed soft stool does not favour the development of piles.

(iii) HIATUS HERNIA

This condition is common in Western man and only attracted attention at the time of the Second World War, which suggests that its prevalence had become greater only recently. It is present in between 10% and 30% of Western middle-aged citizens and is practically unknown in the developing countries. It is not due to pregnancy, otherwise it would be common in rural Africa. It is associated with obesity, diverticulosis and gall-bladder disease, all of which are common in the West, where constipation is a common complaint. Straining of the diaphragm to void hard stools by increasing the intra-abdominal pressure may well be partly responsible for the development of hiatus hernia and the reflux of gastric contents into the lower oesophagus (Burkitt and James, 1973). The association of gallstones, diverticulosis and hiatus hernia is known as Saint's Triad (Muller, 1948).

(d) The Antitoxic Effect of Dietary Fibre

It is well established that the toxic manifestations of various drugs, chemicals, hormones, carcinogens, food additives and other substances can be modified dramatically by the composition of the remainder of the diet. For instance, sodium cyclamate given to rats will retard their growth, cause alopecia and diarrhoea if, at the same time, they are being fed on a purified low-residue diet. It is alarming to note that the dosage of cyclamate required to cause this metabolic upset corresponds to that commonly consumed by human subjects when this chemical was still used commercially as a food additive. This is not to say that cyclamates should continue to be banned while refined sugar is allowed to be sold in unlimited amounts, but is mentioned because it has been shown that these undesirable effects can be counteracted by adding 20% alfalfa meal to this purified diet. The addition of only 10% alfalfa meal or 10% wheat bran considerably lessens both the weight loss and the bowel upset that this chemical causes in rats. Wheat germ, rice bran and cellulose also have a significantly beneficial 'antitoxic' effect. Similarly, sorbitan monostearate (Tween 60) if given to weanling rats in a concentration that proves lethal in only two weeks, can be 'detoxicated' by the addition of alfalfa meal to their purified diet. Not only do these rats, who die on a purified diet and Tween 60, survive, but also gain weight if plant fibre is added to their food (Ershoff, 1960 and 1972).

These and similar experiments leave little doubt that a sufficiency of dietary fibre may protect animals and possibly man from the ill effects of some ingested chemicals. As many food additives are used wherever convenience and processed foods are eaten, and whose long term effects are not known, is it not possible that some modern diseases result from the ingestion of these chemicals? This question becomes even more relevant when it is remembered that any of their harmful effects may be potentiated by the simultaneous ingestion of 'purified' or refined foodstuffs. Two diseases, both of which affect the colon, have been recognized in this century and whose aetiology remains unknown and whose treatment is empirical. These are Crohn's disease and ulcerative colitis. The former is treated surgically if it causes mechanical obstruction and the latter initially is treated medically by drugs whose action is incompletely understood and whose effects are uncertain. Both have the same geographical distribution as diverticular disease and may co-exist or be confused with diverticulitis (Schmidt *et al.*, 1968; Jalan *et al.*, 1970). Hence, the possibility that dietary fibre deficiency may play a direct or indirect part in their causation cannot be ignored. The author prescribes bran in both conditions. Some patients with early ulcerative colitis have been improved clinically in that their stools have become formed and less frequent, but no beneficial effect has been seen in those in the advanced stages of the disease. Nevertheless, it is reasonable to suggest that a long-term trial of wholemeal bread and 'full fibre' might prove instructive and even helpful.

CONCLUSION

Diverticular disease is probably caused by a deficiency of dietary fibre. Hence, it is possible that fibre depletion may help to cause those diseases which have the same epidemiology as diverticulosis. Thus the unabsorbable part of our food should not be ignored by nutritionists as it has been so often in the past.

Fibre is an essential part of our food and the author believes that already there is sufficient evidence to show that the taking of two grams of fibre daily would improve our physical and hence our mental health. This could be added quite easily to our daily bread in the form of bran.

Therapeutically, a high-fibre diet should be prescribed both before and after surgery for complicated diverticular disease and after colonic resections carried out for cancer.

Every process involved in food refining should be investigated as there is no doubt that, in many cases, food technologists and millers do not know what effect their activities have on our health in the long term.

The author is indebted to Professor Nicolas Georgiadis of Athens for a Greek proverb which is particularly apt regarding the removal of fibre from our diet. It refers to anyone who undertakes an activity which he does not understand, such as playing with electricity and getting a shock or keeping bad company and losing both his money and reputation.

The proverb runs, 'He who meddles with the bran gets bitten by the chickens'.

References

ABBE, R. (1914). *Med. Rep.* **86,** 190.

ALLEN, A. W. (1953). *Am. J. Surg.* **86,** 545.

ALMY, T. P., ABBOTT, F. K. and HINKLE, L. E. (1950). *Gastro-enterology* **15,** 95.

ALMY, T. P., HINKLE, L. E., BERLE, B. B. and KERN, F. (1969). *Gastroenterology* **12,** 437.

ALMY, T. P., KERN, F. and TULIN, M. (1949). *Gastroenterology* **12,** 425.

ALVAREZ, W. C. (1958). *Dis. Colon Rectum* **1,** 333.

ANDERSON, D. (1970). Personal Communication.

ANDERSON, L. (1946). *Proc. Staff Meet. Mayo Clin.* **21,** 465.

ARDRAN, G. M. and WYATT, D. G. (1954). *J. Physiol.* **126,** 12.

ARDRAN, G. M. and WYATT, D. G. (1957). *Br. J. Radiol.* **30,** 52.

ARFWIDSSON, S. (1964). *Acta chir. scand.,* Supplement 342.

ARIES, V., CROWTHER, J. S., DRASAR, B. S., MILL, M. J. and WILLIAMS, R. E. O. (1969). *Gut* **10,** 334.

ARNHEIM, E. E. (1940). *Ann. Surg.* **112,** 352.

ATTISHA, R. P. and SMITH, A. N. (1969). *Br. J. Surg.* **56,** 891.

BACON, H. E. and MAGSONOC, C. M. (1964). *Am. J. Surg.* **108,** 830.

BACON, H. E. and SHERMAN, L. F. (1950). *Am. J. Surg.* **80,** 3.

BADO, E. A. (1971). Personal Communication to D. P. Burkitt.

BAILLIE, M. (1797). *Morbid Anatomy,* 2nd edition, London.

BARBORKA, C. J. (1958). *Gastroenterology* **34,** 278.

BARKER, T. C., MCKENZIE, J. C. and YUDKIN, J. (1966). *Our Changing Fare,* McGibbon and Kee, London.

BARLING, S. (1926). *Br. Med. J.* **1,** 322.

BEARD, R. G. and GAZET, J. C. (1961). *Guy's Hosp. Rep.* **110,** 263.

BEARSE, C. (1939). *J. Am. med. Ass.* **113,** 1720.

BEARSE, C. (1946). *J. Am. med. Ass.* **132,** 371.

BECKER, J. L. (1954). *Am. J. dig. Dis.* **19,** 344.

BEER, E. (1904). *Am. J. med. Sci.* **128,** 135.

BELDING, H. H. (1957). *Archs. Surg.* **74,** 571

BELL, C. M. A. and LEWIS, C. B. (1968). *Br. Med. J.* **3,** 587.

BENNETT-JONES, M. J. (1937). *Br. J. Surg.* **25,** 66.

BERMAN, P. M. and KIRSNER, J. B. (1972). *Am. J. dig. Dis.* **17,** 741.

BEVAN, P. G. (1961). *Br. Med. J.* **1**, 400.

BLACK, K. (1953). *Practitioner* **171**, 675.

BLAND-SUTTON, J. (1903). *Lancet* **2**, 1148.

BLAND-SUTTON, J. (1920). *Proc. R. Soc. Med. Section of Surgery* **13**, 64.

BOLES, R. S. and JORDAN, S. M. (1958). *Gastroenterology* **35**, 579.

BOLT, D. E. (1960). *Br. Med. J.* **1**, 832.

BOLT, D. E. (1973). *Ann. R. Coll. Surg. England* **53**, 237.

BOLT, D. E. and HUGHES, L. E. (1966). *Br. Med. J.* **1**, 1205.

BOTSFORD, T. W. and CURTIS, L. E. (1961). *New Engl. J. Med.* **265**, 618.

BOTSFORD, T. W. and ZOLLINGER, R. M. (1969). *Surgery, Gynec. Obstet.* **128**, 1209.

BOTSFORD, T. W., ZOLLINGER, R. M. and HICKS, S. R. (1971). *Am. J. Surg.* **12**, 702.

BOYDEN, A. M. (1950). *Ann. Surg.* **132**, 94.

BREMNER, C. G. and ACKERMAN, L. V. (1970). *Cancer* **26**, 991.

BREWER, G. E. (1907). *Am. J. med. Sci.* **134**, 483.

BRISTOWE, J. S. (1854). *Trans. path. Soc. Lond.* **6**, 191.

BROCKELHURST, J. C., GRIFFITHS, L. L., TAYLOR, G. F., MARKS, J., SCOTT, D. L. and BLACKLEY, J. (1968). *Geront. clin.* **10**, 309.

BRODY, D. A. and QUIGLEY, J. P. (1951), *Meth. med. Res.* **4**, 109 Year Book Publishing Corp., Chicago.

BROWN, D. B. and TOOMEY, W. F. (1960). *Br. J. Surg.* **47**, 485.

BROWN, P. W. and MARCLEY, D. M. (1937). *J. Am. med. Ass.* **109**, 1328.

BROWNE, M. K. (1967). *Clin. Trials J. (London)* **4**, 673.

BROWNE, M. K. and STOLLER, J. L. (1970). *Br. J. Surg.* **57**, 525.

BUIE, L. A. (1939). *New Engl. J. Med.* **221**, 593.

BURKITT, D. P. (1969). *Lancet* **2**, 1229.

BURKITT, D. P. (1971). *Br. J. Surg.* **58**, 695.

BURKITT, D. P. (1973). *Rendic. Gastroenterol.* **5**, 33.

BURKITT, D. P. (1973). *Br. med. J.* **1**, 274.

BURKITT, D. P. and JAMES, P. A. (1973). *Lancet* **2**, 128.

BURKITT, D. P., WALKER, A. R. P. and PAINTER, N. S. (1972). *Lancet* **2**, 1408.

BURKITT, D. P., WALKER, A. R. P. and PAINTER, N. S. (1974). *J. Am. med. Ass.* **229**, 1068.

BYRNE, J. J. and GARICK, E. I. (1971). *Am. J. Surg.* **121**, 379.

CALDER, J. F. (1971). *Br. med. J.* **2**, 654.

CARLSON, A. J. and HOELZEL, F. (1949). *Gastroenterology* **12**, 108.

CARMAN, R. D. (1915). *Am. J. Roentg.* **2**, 652.

CARMAN, R. D. (1915). *Ann. Surg.* **61**, 343.

CASE, J. T. (1915). *Am. J. Roentg.* **2,** 654.

CASE, J. T. (1928). *Am. J. Surg.* **4,** 573.

CHANG, W. Y. M. (1965). *Hawaii med. J.* **24,** 442.

CHAPMAN, D. (1971). Personal Communication.

CHAPMAN, J. (1934). *Annals of intern. Med.* **7,** 1376.

CHAUDHARY, N. A. and TRUELOVE, S. C. (1961). *Gastroenterology* **40,** 1.

CHILDS, PETER (1972). *Br. J. Surg.* **59,** 669.

CHLUMSKY, V. (1899). *Beitr. Klin. Chir.* **25,** 539.

CLEAVE, T. L. (1941). *Br. med. J.* **1,** 461.

CLEAVE, T. L. (1962). 'Peptic Ulcer', John Wright and Sons Ltd, Bristol.

CLEAVE, T. L. (1973). *Lancet* **1,** 1443.

CLEAVE, T. L. (1974). 'The Saccharine Disease', John Wright and Sons Ltd, Bristol.

CLEAVE, T. L., CAMPBELL, G. D. and PAINTER, N. S. (1969). 'Diabetes, Coronary Thrombosis and the Saccharine Disease', 2nd edition, John Wright and Sons Ltd, Bristol.

CLELAND, J. B. (1968). *Br. med. J.* **1,** 579.

COHEN, S. E., CUNNINGHAM, J. R. and SNIERSON, H. (1957). *Archs. Surg.* **75,** 800.

COLCOCK, B. P. (1950). *Surg. Clins. N. Am.* 911.

COLCOCK, B. P. (1971). *Surg. Clins. N. Am.* **51,** 79.

COLCOCK, B. P. (1971). 'Diverticular Disease of the Colon', W. B. Saunders Co., Philadelphia.

CONNELL, A. M. (1961). *Gut* **2,** 175.

CONWAY, F. M. and HITZROT, J. M. (1931). *Ann. Surg.* **94,** 614.

CORRY, D. C. (1963). *Br. med. J.* **2,** 929.

COWGILL, G. R. and ANDERSON, W. E. (1932). *J. Am. med. Ass.* **98,** 1866.

CRIPPS, H. (1888). 'The Passage of Air and Faeces from the Bladder', page 98, Churchill, London.

CRUVEILHIER, J. (1849). 'Traité d'Anatomie Pathologique Générale', **1,** 593.

CUMMINGS, J. H. (1973). *Gut* **14,** 69.

CURTIS, A. C. and KLINE, E. M. (1939). *Archs. intern. Med.* **63,** 54.

DANDEKAR, N. V. and MCCANN, W. J. (1969). *Dis. Colon. Rectum* **12,** 172.

DANIEL, O. (1969). *Proc. R. Soc. Med.* **62,** 811.

DANIEL, O. and SINGH, M. L. (1969). *Br. J. Urol.* **41,** 32.

DAVID, V. C. (1933). *Surgery, Gynec. Obstet.* **56,** 375.

DAWSON, J. L., HANON, I. and ROXBURGH, R. A. (1965). *Br. J. Surg.* **52,** 354.

DEBRAY, C., HARDOUIN, J. P., BESANCON, F. and RAIMBAULT, J. (1961). *Sem. Hôp. Paris* **37**, 1743.
DE QUERVAIN, F. (1914). *Dt. Z. Chir.* **128**, 67.
DE QUERVAIN, F. (1927). *Practitioner* **118**, 352.
DIMOCK, E. (1936). *MD. Thesis*, University of Cambridge.
DONALDSON, R. (1907). *Br. med. J.* **2**, 1705.
DRUMMOND, H. (1917). *Br. J. Surg.* **4**, 407.
DUNN, A. D. and WOOLLEY, P. G. (1911). *Am. J. med. Sci.* **142**, 22.
DUNNING, M. W. F. (1963). *Gut* **4**, 273.

EARLEY, C. M. (1959). *Surgery, Gynec. Obstet.* **108**, 49.
EASTWOOD, M. A. (1969). *Lancet* **2**, 1222.
EASTWOOD, M. A., KIRKPATRICK, J. R., MITCHELL, W. D., BONE, A. and HAMILTON, T. (1973). *Br. med. J.* **4**, 392.
EDEL, M. (1894). *Virchow's Archs.* **138**, 347.
EDWARDS, H. C. (1934). *Lancet* **1**, 221.
EDWARDS, H. C. (1934). *Br. J. Surg.* **22**, 88.
EDWARDS, H. C. (1939). 'Diverticula and Diverticulitis of the Intestine', John Wright and Sons Ltd, Bristol.
EDWARDS, H. C. (1953). *Post-grad. med. J.* **29**, 20.
EDWARDS, H. C. (1954). *Ann. R. Coll. Surg.* **14**, 371.
EGGERS, C. (1941). *Ann. Surg.* **113**, 15.
ENFIELD, C. D. (1924). *Am. J. Roentg.* **12**, 242.
ERSHOFF, B. H. (1960). *J. Nutr.* **70**, 484.
ERSHOFF, B. H. (1972). *Proc. Soc. exp. Biol. Med.* **141**, 857.
EUSEBIO, E. B. and EISENBERG, M. M. (1973). *Am. J. Surg.* **125**, 308.
EWELL, G. H. (1961). *J. int. Coll. Surg.* **36**, 616.

FAGIN, I. D. (1955). *Am. J. dig. Dis.* **22**, 316.
FAIRBANK, T. J. and ROB, C. G. (1947). *Br. J. Surg.* **35**, 105.
FALAIYE, J. M. (1974). *Lancet* **1**, 1002.
FELDMAN, F. and MORRISON, S. (1949). *Am. J. dig. Dis.* **16**, 126.
FIFIELD, L. R. (1927). *Lancet* **1**, 277.
FISCHER, M. H. (1900–1901). *J. exp. Med.* **5**, 332.
FLEISCHMAN (1815). Quoted by SPRIGGS, E. I. and MARXER, O. A. (1925). *Q. Jl. Med.* **19**, 1.
FLEISCHNER, F. G. (1971). *Gastroenterology* **60**, 316.
FLEISCHNER, F. G. and MING, S. C. (1965). *Radiology* **84**, 859.
FLEISCHNER, F. G., MING, S. C. and HENKEN, E. M. (1964). *Radiology* **83**, 859.
FOX, G. and BRADLEY, H. (1958). *Br. med. J.* **2**, 1556.
FOX, J. D., DE WITT, J. and PONKA, J. L. (1959). *Med. Arts Sci.* **13**, 16.
FRAENKEL, G. J. (1954). *Br. J. Surg.* **41**, 643.
FRASER, I. (1933–34). *Br. J. Surg.* **21**, 183.

GIFFIN, H. Z· (1911). *Ann. Surg.* **53**, 533.

GODDING, E. W. (1972). *Lancet* **2**, 1255.

GOODMAN, L. S. and GILMAN, A. (1955). 'The Pharmacological Basis of Therapeutics', 2nd edition, Macmillan, New York.

GORDINIER, H. C. and SAMPSON, J. A. (1906). *J. Am. med. Ass.* **46**, 1585.

GOULSTON, E. (1967). *Br. med. J.* **3**, 359.

GRASER, E. (1899). *München. med. Wschr.* **46**, 721.

GREENE, W. W. (1957). *Am. J. Surg.* **94**, 282.

GRIFFITHS, J. D. (1956). *Ann. R. Coll. Surg.* **19**, 241.

GRIFFITHS, J. D. (1961). *Br. med. J.* **1**, 323.

GROSS, S. D. (1845). 'Elements of Pathological Anatomy', page 554, Blanchard & Lea, Philadelphia.

GROUT, J. L. A. (1949). *Br. J. Radiol.* **22**, 442.

GUY, C. C. and WERELIUS, C. Y. (1952). Surgical Clinics of N. America, 91.

HABERSHON, S. O. (1857). 'Observations on the Alimentary Canal', John Churchill, London.

HAENISCH, F. (1912). *Dt. med. Wschr.* **2**, 1356.

HAMILTON, G. F. (1946). *J. Anat.* **80**, 230.

HANSEMAN, D. (1896). *Virchow's Archs. for Path. and Anat.* **144**, 400.

HARTLEY, R. C. (1964). *Br. J. Surg.* **51**, 45.

HARTWELL, J. A. and CECIL, R. L. (1910). *Am. J. med. Sci.* **140**, 174.

HARVEY, R. F., POMARE, E. W. and HEATON, K. W. (1973). *Lancet* **1**, 1278.

HAVIA, T. (1971). *Acta chir. scand.* Supplement 415.

HAWLEY, P. R. (1973). *Dis. Colon Rectum* **16**, 272.

HAYDEN, E. P. (1940). *New Engl. J. Med.* **222**, 340.

HEALD, R. J. and RAY, J. E. (1971). *Dis. Colon Rectum* **14**, 420.

HEALEY, S. J. and PFEFFER, R. I. (1965). *New Engl. J. Med.* **273**, 1480.

HEATON, K. (1973). *Lancet* **2**, 1418.

HEATON, K. W. and POMARE, E. W. (1974). *Lancet* **1**, 49.

HENDERSON, H. P. (1944). *Br. J. Radiol.* **17**, 197.

HERSCH, R. A. and SCHWABE, A. D. (1963). *Gastroenterology* **45**, 269.

HILL, M. J., CROWTHER, J. S., DRASAR, B. S., HAWKSWORTH, G., ARIES, V. and WILLIAMS, R. E. O. (1971). *Lancet* **1**, 95.

HINTON, J. M., LENNARD-JONES, J. E. and YOUNG, A. L. (1969). *Gut* **10**, 842.

HOARE, E. M. (1970). *Proc-R. Soc. Med.*, Supplement to Vol. 63, page 55.

HODGSON, J. (1972a). *Br. J. Surg.* **59**, 315.

HODGSON, J. (1972b). *Br. med. J.* **3**, 729.

HODGSON, J. (1973). *Dis. Colon Rectum* **16**, 283.

HODGSON, J. (1974). In a paper presented to American Proctologic Society and the Section of Proctology of the Royal Society of Medicine, Washington, 1974.

HOLDSTOCK, D. J., MISIEWICZ, J. J. and WALLACE, S. C. (1969). *Gut* **10**, 19.

HOLMGREN, G. and MYNORS, J. M. (1972). *A. Afr. med. J.* **46**, 918

HORNER, J. L. (1958). *Am. J. dig. Dis.* **3**, 343.

HUGHES, L. E. (1969). *Gut* **10**, 336.

HUGHES, L. E. (1970). *Br. med. J.* **1**, 496.

HUGHES, L. E. (1970). *Gut* **11**, 111.

HUTT, M. S. R. (1970). Personal Communication.

JACKMAN, R. J. and BUIE, L. A. (1943). *J. Am. med. Ass.* **121**, 1144.

JAIN, A. C. (1971). Personal Communication.

JALAN, K. N., WALKER, R. J., PRESCOTT, R. J., BUTTERWORTH, S. T. G., SMITH, A. N. and SIRCUS, W. (1970). *Gut* **11**, 688.

JOHNSON, A. G. (1971). Rendiconte Gastroenterol **3**, 113.

JONES, S. (1859). *Trans. path. Soc. Lond.* **10**, 131.

JUDD, E. S. and MEARS, T. W. (1955). *Archs. Surg.* **70**, 818.

JUDD, E. S. and POLLOCK, L. W. (1924). *Ann. Surg.* **80**, 425.

KEELEY, K. J. (1958). *Med. Proc.* **4**, 281.

KEITH, A. (1910). *Br. med. J.* **1**, 376.

KILLINGBACK, M. J. (1970). *Dis. Colon Rectum* **13**, 444

KIM, E. O. (1964). *New Engl. J. Med.* **271**, 764.

KLEBS, E. (1869). *Handbuch der Pathol. Anat.*, page 271, Berlin 1869.

KOCOUR, E. J. (1937). *Am. J. Surg.* **37**, 433.

KÖHLER, R. (1963). *Acta chir. scand.* **126**, 148.

KUTTY, M. (1970). Personal Communication.

KYLE, J. (1968). *Jl R. Coll. Surg. Edinb.* **13**, 136.

KYLE, J., ADESOLA, A. O., TINCKLER, L. F. and DE BEAUX, J. (1967). *Scand. J. of Gastroenterology* **2**, 77.

LANE, A. (1885). *Guy's Hosp. Rep.* **43**, 48.

LARGE, J. M. (1964). *Lancet* **1**, 413.

LATTO, C., WILKINSON, R. W. and GILMORE, O. J. A. (1973). *Lancet* **1**, 1089.

LAUFMAN, H. (1941). *Surgery, Gynec. Obstet. Int. Abstr. Surg.* **73**, 222.

LENNARD-JONES, J. E., FLETCHER, J. and SHAW, D. G. (1968). *Gut* **9**, 177.

LE ROYER, C. P. and WHITE, B. V. (1948). *New Engl. J. Med.* **239**, 245.

LEVY, J. I. (1972). Personal Communication.

LEWIS, E. E. and SCHNUG, G. E. (1972). *Am. J. Surg.* **124**, 573.

LINDER, J. M. and HOFFMAN, S. (1962). *Surgery, Gynec. Obstet.* **114,** 755.

LINEBACK, P. E. (1925). *Am. J. Anat.* **36,** 357.

LLOYD-DAVIES, O. V. (1953). *Proc. R. Soc. Med.* **46,** 407.

LOCKHART-MUMMERY, H. E. (1949). *Br. J. Surg.* **36,** 319.

LOCKHART-MUMMERY, H. E. (1958). *Proc. R. Soc. Med.* **51,** 1032.

LOCKHART-MUMMERY, J. P. (1930). *Lancet* **1,** 231.

LOCKHART-MUMMERY, J. P. (1938). *Lancet* **2,** 1401.

LOOMIS, A. L. (1870). *N.Y. med. Record* **4,** 497 (quoted by Hartwell and Cecil, 1910).

LUMSDEN, K. and TRUELOVE, S. C. (1959). *Br. J. Radiol.* **32,** 517.

LUNDING, K. (1935). *Acta med. scand.,* Supplement 72.

LYON, A. S. (1948). *Ann. Surg.* **127,** 398.

MCCANCE, R. A. and WIDDOWSON, E. M. (1956). 'Breads, White and Brown', Pitman Medical Press, London.

MCCUNE, W. S., IOVINE, V. M. and MILLER, D. (1957). *Ann. Surg.* **145,** 683.

MACGREGOR, A. B., ABERNETHY, B. C. and THOMSON, J. W. W. (1970). *Jl R. Coll. Surg., Edinb.* **15,** 137.

MACLAREN, I. F. (1957). *Jl R. Coll. Surg. Edinb.* **3,** 129.

MADDEN, J. L. (1966). *Dis. Colon Rectum* **9,** 413.

MADDEN, J. L. and TAN, P. T. (1961). *Surgery Gynec. Obstet.* **113,** 646.

MANOUSSOS, O. N., TRUELOVE, S. C. and LUMSDEN, K. (1967). *Br. med. J.* **3,** 762.

MAYO, C. W. and BLUNT, C. P. (1950). *Surgery Gynec. Obstet.* **91,** 612.

MAYO, C. W. and BLUNT, C. P. (1950). *Surg. Clins. N. Am.* 1005.

MAYO, W. J. (1930). *Ann. Surg.* **92,** 739.

MAYO, W. J., WILSON, L. B. and GIFFEN, H. Z. (1907). *Surgery Gynec. Obstet.* **5,** 8.

MIANGOLARRA, C. J. (1961). *Ann. Surg.* **153,** 861.

MIELKE, J. E., BECKER, K. L. and GROSS, J. B. (1965). *Gastroenterology* **48,** 379.

MILES, W. E. (1920). *Proc. R. Soc. Med. Section of Surgery* **13,** 84.

MILLER, D. W. and WICHERN, W. A. (1971). *Am. J. Surg.* **121,** 536.

MILLER, R. (1971). Personal Communication.

MOORE, H. D. (1969). *Dis. Colon Rectum* **12,** 22.

MORSON, B. C. (1963). *Br. J. Radiol.* **36,** 385.

MORTON, J. J. (1946). *Ann. Surg.* **124,** 725.

MOYNIHAN, B. G. A. (1907). *Br. med. J.* **2,** 1381.

MOYNIHAN, B. G. A. (1907). *Edin. med. J.* **21,** 228.

MUIR, E. G. (1966). *Lancet* **1,** 195.

MULLER, C. J. B. (1948). *S. Afr. med. J.* **22**, 376.

NOER, R. J. (1955). *Ann. Surg.* **141**, 674.
NOER, R. J. (1959). *Surgery* **45**, 1029.

OLSEN, W. R. (1968). *Am. J. Surg.* **115**, 247.
OSHNER, H. C. and BARGEN, J. A. (1935). *Ann. intern. Med.* **9**, 282.

PACE, J. L. and WILLIAMS, I. (1969). *Gut* **10**, 352.
PAINTER, N. S. (1962). Master of Surgery Thesis, University of London.
PAINTER, N. S. (1964). *Ann. R. Coll. Surg. of England* **34**, 98.
PAINTER, N. S. (1967). *Am. J. dig. Dis.* **12**, 222.
PAINTER, N. S. (1968). *Br. med. J.* **3**, 475.
PAINTER, N. S. (1969). *Lancet* **2**, 586.
PAINTER, N. S. (1970). Disease-a-Month, June issue Year Book, Medical Publishers Inc., Chicago.
PAINTER, N. S. (1970). *Proc. R. Soc. Med.*, Supplement to Vol. 63, page 144.
PAINTER, N. S. (1972a). *Br. med. J.* **2**, 46.
PAINTER, N. S. (1972b). *Nutrition, Lond.* **26**, 95.
PAINTER, N. S. (1972c). *Rendic. Gastroenterol.* **4**, 35.
PAINTER, N. S. (1973). *Update* **6**, 1821.
PAINTER, N. S., ALMEIDA, A. Z. and COLEBOURNE, K. W. (1972). *Br. med. J.* **2**, 137.
PAINTER, N. S. and BURKITT, D. P. (1971). *Br. med. J.* **2**, 450.
PAINTER, N. S. and TRUELOVE, S. C. (1963). *Br. med. J.* **2**, 33.
PAINTER, N. S. and TRUELOVE, S. C. (1964a). *Gut* **5**, 201.
PAINTER, N. S. and TRUELOVE, S. C. (1964b). *Gut* **5**, 207.
PAINTER, N. S. and TRUELOVE, S. C. (1964c). *Gut* **5**, 365.
PAINTER, N. S. and TRUELOVE, S. C. (1964d). *Gut* **5**, 369.
PAINTER, N. S., TRUELOVE, S. C., ARDRAN, G. M. and TUCKEY, M. (1965a), *Gastroenterology* **49**, 169.
PAINTER, N. S., TRUELOVE, S. C., ARDRAN, G. M. and TUCKEY, M. (1965b). *Gut* **6**, 57.
PARKS, T. G. (1968). *Proc. R. Soc. Med.* **61**, 30.
PARKS, T. G. (1969). *Br. med. J.* **4**, 639.
PARKS, T. G. (1969). *Br. med. J.* **4**, 642.
PARKS, T. G. (1970). *Gut* **11**, 121.
PARKS, T. G. (1973). *Proc. R. Soc. Med.* **66**, 681.
PARKS, T. G. and CONNELL, A. M. (1969). *Gut* **10**, 538.
PARKS, T. G. and CONNELL, A. M. (1970). *Br. J. Surg.* **57**, 775.
PARKS, T. G. and CONNELL, A. M. (1972). *Rendic. Gastroenterol* **4**, 12.
PARKS, T. G., CONNELL, A. M., GOUGH, A. D. and COLE, J. Y. (1970). *Br. med. J.* **2**, 136

PATEL, M. (1911). *Rev. de Med. de Paris* (quoted by Spriggs and Marxer, 1925).

PATTERSON, C. O. (1951). *Gastroenterology* **18**, 201.

PATTON, R. J. (1953). *Ann. Surg.* **66**, 410.

PAYLOR, D. K. (1973). *Lancet* **1**, 1394.

PECK, D. A., LAMBERT, R. and WAITE, V. C. (1968). *Dis. Colon Rectum* **11**, 49.

PEMBERTON, J. DE J., BLACK, B. M. and MAINO, C. R. (1947). *Surgery Gynec. Obstet.* **85**, 523.

PICKARD, R. G. (1972). *Br. J. Surg.* **59**, 642.

PIEPMEYER, J. L. (1974). *Am. J. clin. Nutr.* **2**, 106.

PLENYVANIT, P. (1972). Personal Communication.

PLUMLEY, P. F. and FRANCIS, B. (1973). *J. Am. diet. Ass.* **6**, 527.

POIRIER, P. and CHARPEY, A. (1914). *Traité d'Anat. Humaine* vol. 4, p. 303.

POMARE, E. W. and HEATON, K. W. (1973). *Br. med. J.* **4**, 262.

POMARE, E. W. and HEATON, K. W. (1973). *Gut* **14**, 885.

PONKA, J. L., FOX, J. D. and BRUSH, B. E. (1959). *Anchs. Surg.* **19**, 373.

PONKA, J. L. and HAYS, T. V. (1972). *Sth. med. J.* **65**, 985.

POTIER, F. (1912). *Bull. Soc. Anat., Paris* **87**, 29.

POWER, D'ARCY (1906). *Br. med. J.* **2**, 1171.

QUINN, W. C. (1961). *Ann. Surg.* **153**, 851.

RAMANATH, H. F., HINSHAW, J. R. (1971). *Anchs. Surg.* **103**, 311.

RANKIN, F. W. (1930). *Surgery, Gynec. Obstet.* **50**, 594.

RANKIN, F. W. and BROWN, P. W. (1930). *Surgery Gynec. Obstet.* **50**, 836.

RAO, D. B. and KATARIA, M. S. (1967). *Br. med. J.* **3**, 238.

REID, D. R. K. (1951). *Br. J. Surg.* **39**, 76.

REILLY, M. (1964). *Proc. R. Soc. Med.* **57**, 576.

REILLY, M. (1966). *Br. J. Surg.* **53**, 859.

REILLY, M. (1969). *Proc. R. Soc. Med.* **62**, 715.

REILLY, M. (1971). 'Modern Trends in Surgery', Vol. 13, Butterworths, London.

ROBERTS, J. L. (1908). *Br. med. J.* **1**, 1174.

ROBERTSON, J. (1972). *Nature, Lond.* **238**, 290.

RODKEY, G. V. and WELCH, C. E. (1959). 'Diseases of Colon and Rectum', Vol. 2, page 633, W. B. Saunders, Co. Philadelphia.

RODKEY, G. V. and WELCH, C. E. (1969). *Am. J. Surg.* **117**, 265.

ROKITANSKY, C. (1849). 'A Manual of Pathological Anatomy', Vol. 2, page 48, The Sydenham Society, London.

ROWLANDS, B. (1951). *Br. med. J.* **2**, 29.

ROXBURGH, R. A., DAWSON, J. L. and YEO, R. (1968). *Br. med. J.* **3,** 465.
RYAN, P. (1958). *Br. J. Surg.* **45,** 611.
RYAN, P. (1965). *Br. J. Surg.* **52,** 85.

SAGAR, S. (1973). *Br. J. clin. Pract.* **27,** 145.
SANDERSON, F. R. (1954). *Med. Ann. Distr. Columbia* **23**(10)**,** 563.
SCHAPIRA, A., LEICHTLING, J. J., WOLF, B. S., MARSHAK, R. H. and JANOWITZ, H. D. (1958). *Am. J. dig. Dis.* **3,** 351.
SCHLOTTHAUER, H. L. (1946). *Ann. Surg.* **124,** 497.
SCHMIDT, G. T., LENNARD-JONES, J. E., MORSON, B. C. and YOUNG, A. C. (1968). *Gut* **9,** 7.
SCHOWENGERDT, C. G., HEDGES, G. R., YAW, P. B. and ALTEMEIER, W. A. (1969), *Archs. Surg.* **98,** 500.
SHORT, A. R. (1920). *Br. J. Surg.* **8,** 171.
SIMPSON, I. (1972), Personal Communication.
SLACK, W. W. (1962). *Br. Surg.* **50,** 185.
SLACK, W. W. (1969). *Proc. R. Soc. Med.*, Supplement to Vol. 63, page 49.
SLESINGER, E. G. (1930). *Lancet* **1,** 1325.
SMILEY, D. F. (1966). *Am. J. Surg.* **111,** 431.
SMITH, A. N. (1973). In a paper presented to the Annual Meeting of the Association of Surgeons at Aberdeen, April 1973.
SMITH, A. N., ATTISHA, R. P. and BALFOUR, T. (1969). *Br. J. Surg.* **56,** 895.
SMITH, A. N., ATTISHA, R. P. and CLARKE, S. (1971). *Am. J. dig. Dis.* **16,** 728.
SMITH, A. N., GIANNAKOS, V. and CLARKE, S. (1971). *Jl R. Coll. Surg. Edinb.* **16,** 276.
SMITH, C. C. and CHRISTENSEN, W. R. (1959). *Am. J. Roentg.* **82,** 996.
SMITH, N. D. (1951). *Am. J. Surg.* **82,** 583.
SMITHWICK, R. M. (1942). *Ann. Surg.* **115,** 969.
SMITHWICK, R. M. (1960). *Am. J. Surg.* **99,** 192.
SOLOMON, A. (1971). Personal Communication.
SPRIGGS, E. I. (1920). *Proc. R. Soc. Med.* **13,** Section of Surgery, page 65.
SPRIGGS, E. I. and MARXER, O. A. (1925). *Q. Jl Med.* **19,** 1.
SPRIGGS, E. I. and MARXER, O. A. (1927). *Lancet* **1,** 1067.
STAUNTON, M. D. (1962). *Br. med. J.* **1,** 916.
STEMMERMAN, G. N. (1970). *Archs. envir. Hlth.* **20,** 266.
STEMMERMAN, G. N. and YATANI, R. (1973). *Cancer* **31,** 1260.
STOUT, A. P. (1923). *Archs. Surg.* **6,** 793.
STRENGER, G. (1957). *Am. J. Surg.* **94,** 577.
SUDSUKI, K. (1900). *Arch. klin. Chir.* **61,** 708.

TAGART, R. E. B. (1953). *Br. J. Surg.* **40,** 437.
TAGART, R. E. B. (1969). *Br. J. Surg.* **56,** 417.
TAYLOR, G. and LAKIN, C. E. (1910). *Lancet* **1,** 495.
TAYLOR, G. F. (1973). Personal Communication.
TAYLOR, R. S. (1966). *Br. J. Surg.* **53,** 947.
TELLING, W. H. M. (1908). *Lancet* **1,** 843.
TELLING, W. H. M. (1920). *Proc. R. Soc. Med.* **13,** 55.
TELLING, W. H. M. and GRUNER, O. C. (1917). *Br. J. Surg.* **4,** 468.
TEMPLETON, A. C. (1970). Personal Communication.
THOMPSON, G. F. and FOX, P. F. (1944). *Am. J. Surg.* **66,** 280.
THOMPSON, H. R. (1959). *Postgrad. med. J.* **35,** 86.
TODD, I. P. (1955). *Ann. R. Coll. Surg. of England,* **16,** 118.
TORSOLI, A., CRUCIOLI, V. and YOUNG, A. C. (1969). *Rendic. Gastroenterol.* **1,** 195.
TOVEY, F. L. (1971). *Trop. geogr. Med.* **24,** 107.
TOVEY, F. L. (1972). *J. Christ. med. Ass., India* **47,** 312.
TROWELL, H. C. (1960). 'Non-infective Diseases in Africa', Arnold, London.
TROWELL, H. C. (1972). *Eur. J. clin. biol. Res.* **17,** 345.
TROWELL, H. C. (1972). *Atherosclerosis* **16,** 138.
TROWELL, H. C. (1974). *Lancet* **1,** 503.
TROWELL, H. C., PAINTER, N.S. and BURKITT, D. P. (1974). *Am. J. dig. Dis.* **19,** 864.
TURNER, G. G. (1920). *Proc. R. Soc. med.* **13,** Section of Surgery, 68.

ULIN, A. W., SOKOLIC, I. H. and THOMPSON, C. (1959). *Ann. intern. Med.* **50,** 1395.

VAUGHAN-WILLIAMS, E. M. and STREETER, D. H. P. (1950). *Br. J. Pharmac.* **5,** 584.
VIRCHOW, R. (1853). *Arch. path. Anat. Physiol.* **5,** 335.
VOIGTEL, F. G. (1804). Handbuch der Pathologischen Anatomie, Vol. 2, Halle, 1804.

WALKER, A. R. P. (1961). *S. Afr. med. J.* **35,** 114.
WALKER, A. R. P. (1964). *Circulation* **29,** 1.
WALKER, A. R. P. (1972). *Am. J. clin. Nutr.* **21,** 518.
WALKER, A. R. P. (1974). *Ann. intern. Med.* **80,** 663.
WALKER, A. R. P. (1974). *Am. J. clin. Nutr.* In the press.
WALKER, A. R. P. and WALKER, B. F. (1969). *Br. med. J.* **2,** 238.
WALKER, A. R. P., WALKER, B. F. and RICHARDSON, B. D. (1970). *Br. med. J.* **3,** 48.
WALKER, A. R. P., WALKER, B. F., RICHARDSON, B. D. and WORLORD, A. (1973). *Postgrad. med. J.* **49,** 243.

WAPNICK, S. and LEVIN, L. (1971). *Br. med. J.* **3**, 115.
WATKINS, G. L. and OLIVER, G. A. (1966). *Archs. Surg.* **92**, 928.
WATT, J. and MARCUS, R. (1964). *J. Path. Bact.* **88**, 97.
WAUGH, J. M. and WALT, A. J. (1957). *Surgery, Gynec. Obstet.* **105**, 690.
WAUGH, J. M. and WALT, A. J. (1959). *Surg. Clins. N. Am.* **39**, 1281.
WEINGARTEN, M., VENET, L. and VICTOR, M. B. (1959). *Gastroenterology* **36**, 642.
WELCH, C. E., ALLEN, A. W. and DONALDSON, G. A. (1953). *Ann. Surg.* **138**, 332.
WELCH, C. E. and RODKEY, G. V. (1956). *Surgery* **39**, 712.
WELLS, C. (1949). *Br. J. Radiol.* **22**, 449.
WHELAN, C. S., FURCINITTI, J. F. and LAVAREDDA, C. (1971). *Am. J. Surg.* **121**, 374.
WILKINS, J. L., HARDCASTLE, J. D., MANN, C. V. and KAUFMAN, L. (1970). *Br. med. J.* **1**, 793.
WILLARD, J. H. and BOCKUS, H. L. (1936). *Am. J. dig. Dis. Nutr.* **3**, 580.
WILLIAMS, I. (1963). *Br. J. Radiol.* **36**, 393.
WILLIAMS, I. (1967). *Radiology* **89**, 401.
WILSON, R. R. (1950). *Br. J. of Surg.* **38**, 65.
WOLF, A. E. M. (1931). *Lancet* **1**, 525.
WRIGHT, D. H. (1970). Personal Communication.

YAZAWA, C. (1973). At Meeting of International Society of Colon and Rectal Surgeons, Rhodes, 1973.
YOUNG, J. M. and HOWARTH, M. B. (1954). *Ann. of Surg.* **140**, 128.
YUDKIN, J. (1972). 'Pure, White and Deadly', Dovis-Poynter Ltd, London.

Index